MOLLY FOX'S STEP ON IT

MOLLY FOX'S STEP ON IT

MOLLY FOX
AND
DEBORAH BROIDE

Photographs by Robin Rice

AVON BOOKS NEW YORK

George W. Stuart

—M.F.

For Don and Alex with love

—D.L.B.

A NOTE OF CAUTION

Before beginning this, or any other, exercise program, it is advisable to obtain the approval and recommendations of your physician. While you're on this, or any, exercise program, it is advisable to visit your physician for periodic monitoring. This program is intended for people of all ages in good health.

AVON BOOKS
A division of
The Hearst Corporation
105 Madison Avenue
New York, New York 10016

Copyright © 1991 by Molly Fox and Deborah Broide
Cover photograph and all interior photographs by Robin Rice
Book design by Richard Oriolo
Published by arrangement with the authors
Library of Congress Catalog Card Number: 91-6554
ISBN: 0-380-76370-2

Library of Congress Cataloging in Publication Data:
Fox, Molly.
  [Step on it]
  Molly Fox's step on it / Molly Fox and Deborah Broide ; photographs by Robin Rice.
    p.   cm.
  1. Exercise. 2. Aerobic exercises. I. Broide, Deborah. II. Title.
GV481.F66 1991
613.7'1—dc20   91-6554
                                                           CIP

First Avon Books Trade Printing: May 1991

AVON TRADEMARK REG. U.S. PAT OFF. AND IN OTHER COUNTRIES, MARCA REGISTRADA, HECHO EN U.S.A.

Printed in the U.S.A.

ARC 10 9 8 7 6 5 4 3 2 1

Acknowledgments

First, I want to thank Deborah Broide for the idea and faith to get this book launched. Without her this book would never be. Thanks again to Robin Rice, whose photographs grace these pages, and to John Giswold and Kacy Duke, whose faces and spirits are contained in this book. Special thanks to Debra for love and emotional support—it helps more than you know—and to Liza Fox for being the most beautiful daughter on the planet. Finally to Rebecca Thomas and all the staff at the Molly Fox Studio, I love you all, thank you again and again, for without you there is no first step.

—M.F.

For their help and support I would like to thank Don Rieck, Marilyn and Harry Broide, Bruce Sinofsky, Harriet Bell, Lisa Berkowitz, Julie Amper, Robin Rice, John Giswold, Kacy Duke, Judith Riven and Mark Gompertz of Avon, and Tamilee Webb, author of Tamilee Webb's Original Rubber Band Workout, who introduced me to the world of fitness all those years ago. I would also like to thank my local aerobics studio, The Body Shop in Montclair, N.J., for their excellent classes (a haven away from my computer), and for the interest and encouragement of the instructors and students during the writing of this book. Finally, and most genuinely, I would like to sing the praises of Molly Fox—a knowledgeable, vivacious, enthusiastic, and most important, inspiring woman, who has made fitness fun for so many people.

—D.L.B.

Contents

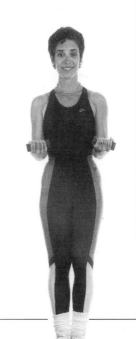

WELCOME TO MOLLY FOX'S STEP ON IT

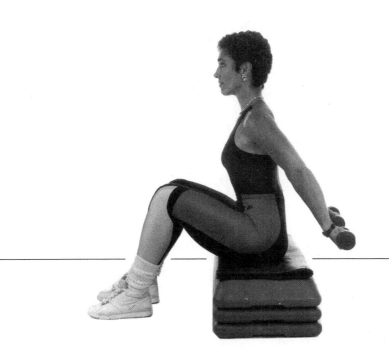

What Is Step On It?

Step On It is a high-intensity low-impact aerobic workout for all fitness levels. The principle behind Step On It is simple—step up and down on a platform while simultaneously performing upper torso body-building movements. Light weights—one or two pounds—may be added for extra upper body toning. The program works every major muscle group in the lower body, while also training the upper body. It not only shapes, tightens, and defines muscles, but also it burns the maximum amount of fat. Step On It is especially good for extra leg toning, including buttocks, quadriceps (the front of the thighs), and hamstrings (the back of the thighs).

The step is also used for performing strengthening and conditioning exercises.

How Safe Is Step On It?

Step On It combines the best of high- and low-impact aerobics. While high-impact aerobics may lead to an increase in injuries, especially in the lower leg, foot, and knees, low-impact aerobics, although safer, may lack intensity and thus burn less fat. Step On It is similar to walking three miles per hour, while the cardiorespiratory fitness benefits and calorie burning are comparable to running at seven miles per hour. Best of all, Step On It is easy on the legs, knees, and feet—there is no bouncing. The consistent movement in a Step On It program (each step is the same height) makes the workout less jarring than other aerobics programs. The step movements are at a comfortable 120 beats-per-minute pace. Of course, as in any exercise program, you should check with your doctor before participating in the activity.

Can I Use My Front Steps Instead of the Step Equipment?

Many of the steps in Molly Fox's Step On It program may be modified for home step use. However, be sure that your entire foot fits on the home step. Over the Top, Propulsion, and Off the End steps are *not* suitable for home step use. You may use a mat or a rug for the conditioning section of the program instead of a step.

Music

Step to the music! Fun music with the right beat makes step training even more invigorating and effective. The tempo should be 120 beats per minute (this is a little slower than the music used in a regular aerobics class). You can either buy a specially mixed aerobics step tape (available at fitness stores or through fitness magazines), create your own tape, or turn on your local top-forty station and step to the songs of Madonna, Taylor Dane, Paula Abdul, Janet Jackson, Donna Summer, Technotronics, or any number of rap groups. Many of these artists' music comply with the 120-beats-per-minute requirement.

Getting Started

Novice—New to Exercise

Begin with the step (most are four inches high) with one bracelet under each side of the step (the step now becomes six inches high). If this is too high, remove one of the bracelets and just use the step.

Perform all the warm-up exercises. Then do ten minutes of the step program. You must start Step On It slowly, gradually building up strength in your leg muscles. You may add ten minutes of walking to increase your aerobic activity. After four to six weeks at your current step program you should be able to increase your step time to twenty minutes. Four to six weeks later you may once again extend your step time to thirty minutes. After you have mastered thirty minutes, you may add another bracelet on each side of the step (you now have an eight-inch step). Stay there for at least six weeks; then if desired, increase the step height again. The higher the step, the more difficult the workout. If you feel any knee pain while exercising, remove a bracelet and continue from the lesser height. You might have progressed too soon.

Beginner Stepper—Already Exercising but New to Step On It

For a carefree transition to Step On It, add or substitute ten minutes of step to your regular exercise program. You may start with either one or two bracelets under the step and slowly increase both the length of exercise time and the height of the step. Your ultimate step time goal is twenty to forty minutes.

Intermediate/Advanced Stepper—Already Been Stepping On It for Several Months

You may design the perfect workout for yourself by varying the step height and the length of time on the step. One day you might try a ten- or twelve-inch step for thirty minutes. Another day, try an eight-inch step for forty minutes. At the intermediate or advanced stage you may use one- or two-pound weights for more upper body definition. Add weights slowly; use for ten minutes at first, then keep increasing the length of time.

How Often Should I Step On It?

The American College of Sports Medicine recommends twenty to fifty minutes of cardiovascular training, three to five times a week, at 65 to 85 percent of your maximum heart rate.

To target your appropriate intensity level, you must first assess your resting heart rate by taking your pulse. To locate your pulse take your index and middle fingers and place them on the outside of your eye, near the temple, then draw the fingers down to your neck and press lightly. If you can't find your pulse this way, try pressing the index finger and the middle finger on the inside of the wrist, with your palm facing up, and press lightly. For your resting heart rate count the beats for sixty seconds. After you have determined your heart rate look at the left of the chart to find the number closest to your age. Then look at the top column to find your resting heart rate. Follow the two numbers down to where they intersect and you will find your aerobic target

Target Heart Rate Zones*
(numbers in boxes are pulse counts per ten seconds)

		Resting Heart Rate								
		50	55	60	65	70	75	80	85	90
	15	24-28	24-27	25-28	25-28	25-29	26-29	26-29	26-29	27-29
	20	23-27	23-27	24-28	25-28	25-28	25-28	25-28	26-29	26-29
	25	23-26	23-27	24-27	24-27	24-27	25-28	25-28	25-28	26-28
	30	22-26	23-26	23-26	23-26	24-27	24-27	24-27	25-27	25-28
	35	22-25	22-25	23-26	23-26	23-26	24-26	24-26	24-27	25-27
	40	21-25	21-24	22-25	22-25	23-25	23-26	23-26	24-26	24-26
Age	45	21-24	21-24	21-24	21-24	22-25	23-25	23-25	23-25	23-26
	50	20-23	21-24	21-24	21-24	22-24	22-25	22-25	23-25	23-25
	55	20-23	20-23	20-23	21-23	21-24	21-24	22-24	22-24	22-24
	60	19-22	20-22	20-22	20-23	21-24	21-23	21-23	22-24	22-24
	65	19-21	19-22	19-22	20-22	20-22	20-23	21-23	21-23	21-23
	70	18-21	19-21	19-21	19-21	20-22	20-22	20-22	21-22	21-22
	75	18-20	18-20	18-21	19-21	19-21	19-21	20-21	20-22	20-22
	80	17-20	18-20	18-20	18-20	19-20	19-21	19-21	20-21	20-21

*From *If It Hurts Don't Do It*, by Peter Francis and Lorna Francis, Prima Publisher, CA, 1988.

heart rate. After you are finished with the aerobic section of *Step On It*, take a ten-second pulse and compare your number to your target heart rate on the chart. If your number is lower than it is supposed to be, you may increase your range of motion or increase your step height. If it is higher, decrease your intensity by excluding arm movements and range of motion or lowering your step height. After the cool down, take another resting heart rate pulse (for sixty seconds) to make sure that you're sufficiently recovered.

In order to increase the step height a "bracelet" is added on either side of the step platform. A bracelet is hard plastic, and blocklike; bracelets can be stacked on top of each other like Legos (thus increasing the step height).

Determining Step Height

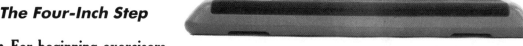

The Four-Inch Step

- For beginning exercisers

- For pregnant exercisers (with a doctor's permission)

- For overweight exercisers

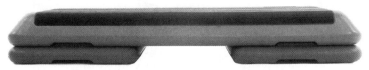

The Six-Inch Step

- For beginning stepper—a person who has been exercising but is new to Step On It

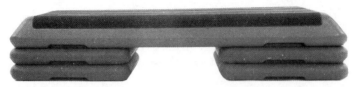

The Eight-Inch Step

- For the intermediate stepper—a person who is in good condition and who has been stepping for eight weeks

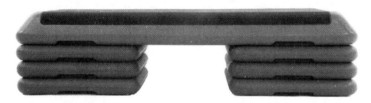

The Ten-Inch Step

- For the advanced stepper—a person who is a skilled and conditioned stepper. The skills include strength, balance, proper alignment, and endurance.

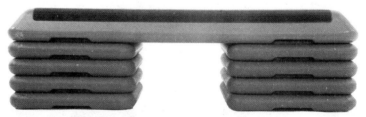

The Twelve-Inch Step

- For the athlete—a person who is masterful at stepping. This stepper is conditioned like an athlete with very strong leg and abdominal muscles.

SAFETY TIPS

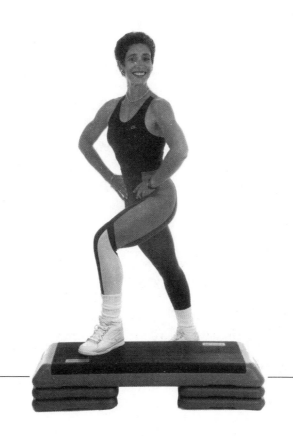

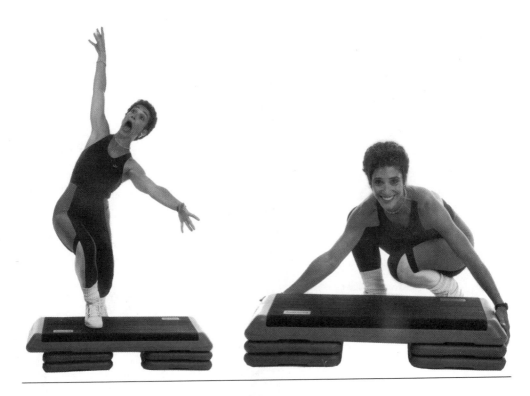

1.

Before you Step On It be sure that the bracelets are snapped in securely. Line up the corners of the bracelets with the corners of the steps.

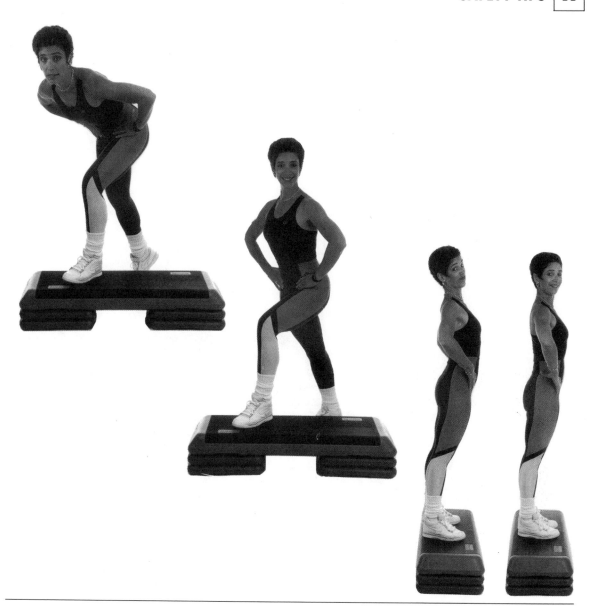

2.

A full body lean is necessary when you step up. Never lean over from the back—it's hard on your back and unnecessary. Your body weight goes with you. Don't arch your back either.

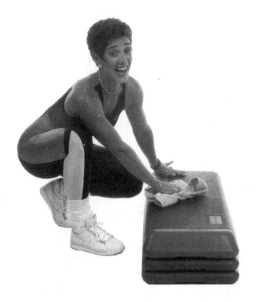

3.

Keep a towel handy to wipe up the sweat; the step itself can get slippery. You'll sweat a lot more in a Step On It program than in a regular class—so take a moment and wipe up the sweat.

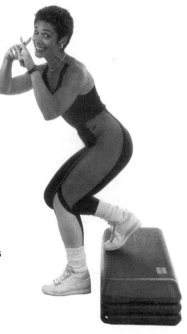

4.

Never step forward *off* the step. Always step back off, facing the step.

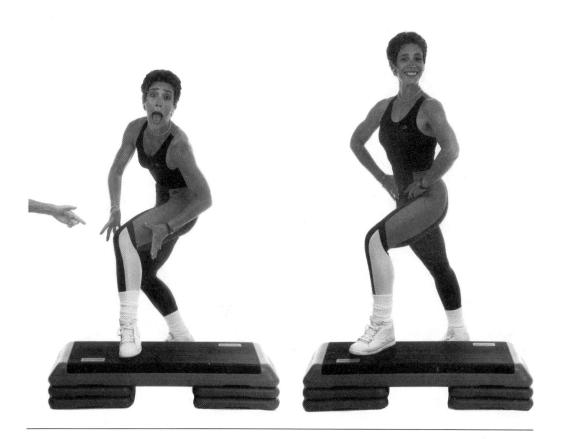

5.

Remember to keep your knees over your toes and line your knees and toes up with your hips on all diagonal turning steps. Step up with the foot that is closest to the step.

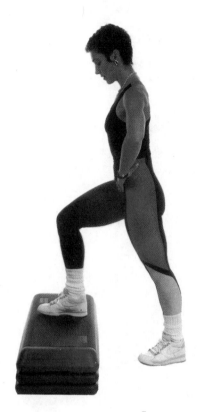

6.

Always step to the center of the step. As a novice or beginner be sure to check your foot on the step every few steps. Be sure it is still in the center of the step.

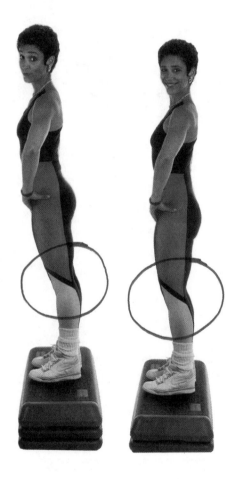

7.

Never lock your knees. Always keep your knees soft.

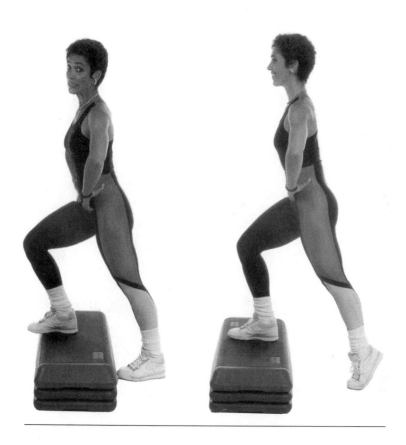

8.

Never overshoot your step (do not let your foot dangle off the edge of the step).
Step directly to the center with the entire foot on the step.

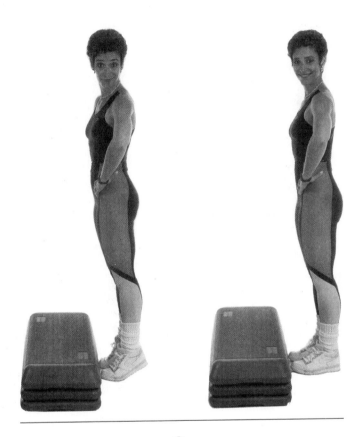

9.

Never land on the balls of the feet. When stepping down, land on the *ball* of the foot, and follow through to the *heel*; get the entire foot down, except when lunging or doing propulsion steps (here just the ball of the foot touches).

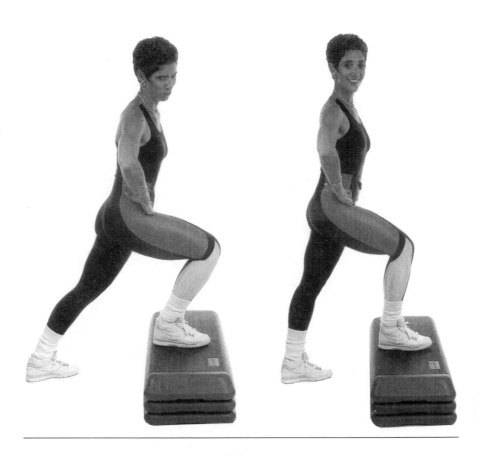

10.

Never flex your knee beyond ninety degrees. Check your knee flexion from the back of the knee. If you are short, be sure that your step is not too high (regardless of your physical fitness condition).

11.

Keep your feet fairly close to the step when stepping down.

12.

Never run on the step—running increases the impact on your foot and lower leg. Always relax and walk.

13.

Always drink water before, during, and after exercise. As a stepper you will sweat a lot. Be sure to replenish your body's natural fluids by drinking water.

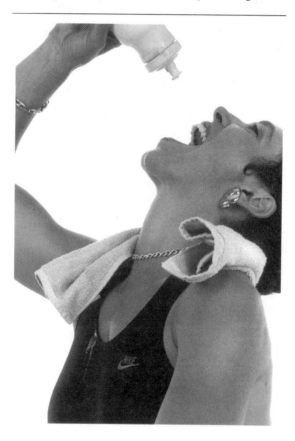

WARM-UPS

A good warm-up is an essential component in any exercise program. A warm-up not only literally warms up the joints, muscles, ligaments, and tendons but also it raises the core temperature of the body. The warm-up program of Molly Fox's Step On It prepares you for the specific sport of stepping.

You will begin with two to four minutes of rhythmic or continuous movement, followed by six to eight minutes of static (no bouncing) stretches. Hold each stretch for eight to ten seconds—relax into the stretch. In the movement section of the warm-up, use full range of motion. After the warm-up phase your breath should be taxed—you are beginning to get to work.

Body Awareness
(Do each exercise in sequence)

1. Breather

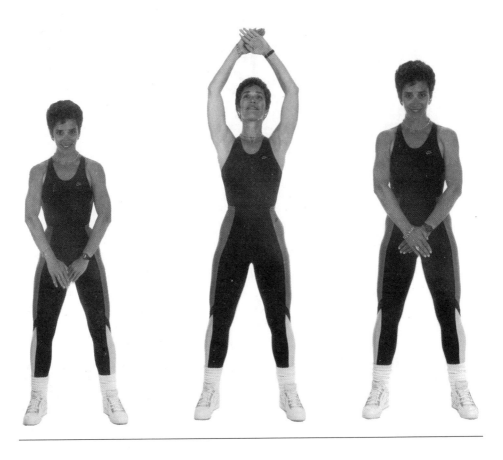

1.

Stand with your feet hip width apart. Put your arms down in front of your body.

2.

Inhale as you extend your arms out and up. Look up toward your hands. Perform in four counts.

3.

Exhale as you lower your arms back to the starting position. Perform in four counts.

4.

Repeat this exercise four times.

Do not lean or arch your back.

2. Head Circles

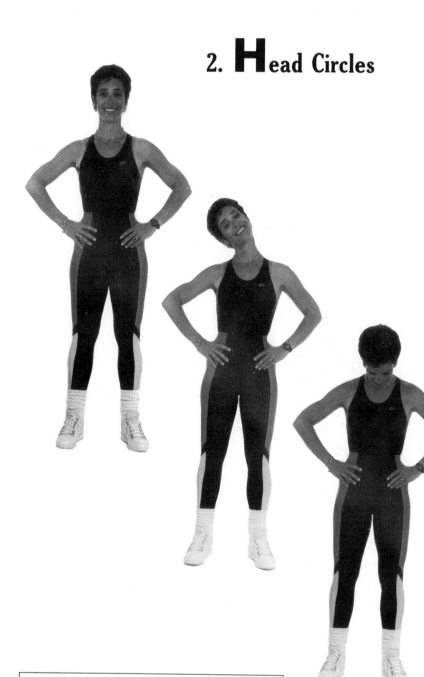

1.

Stand with your feet hip width apart. Keep your knees soft; pull your abdominals in; put your hands on your hips.

2.

Drop your right ear to your right shoulder in four counts.

3.

Drop your chin to your chest in four counts.

4.

Drop your left ear to your left shoulder in four counts.

5.

Return to the beginning position.

6.

Repeat four times.

Do not drop your head back.

3. **S**houlder rolls

1.

Stand with your feet hip width apart. Keep your knees soft; pull your abdominals in; roll your shoulders forward.

2.

Continue rolling in a circle as shoulders roll up.

3.

Shoulders roll back.

4.

Return to resting position.

5.

Do this two times, then reverse circles.

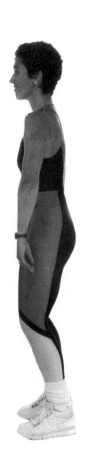
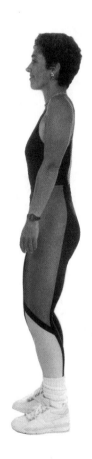
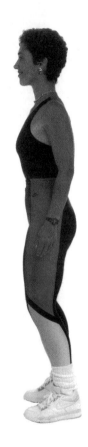

4. Upper Back

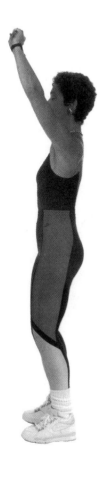

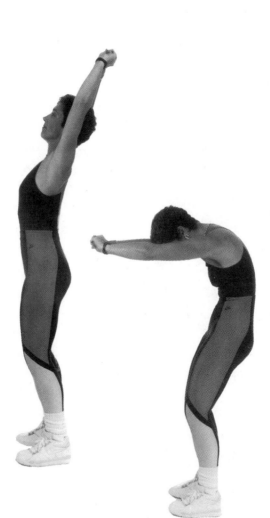

1.

Stand with your feet hip width apart. Keep your knees soft, your abdominals pulled in, and your buttocks squeezed. Lift your arms up over your head with your fingers laced.

2.

Inhale and stretch your arms back while lifting your chest up as you look up. Do this in four counts.

3.

Exhale and stretch and reach your arms forward. Keep your abdominals in and your buttocks squeezed as you stretch your upper back. Do this in four counts.

4.

Repeat four times.

Do not lean back. Think "lift up."

5. **L**ower back

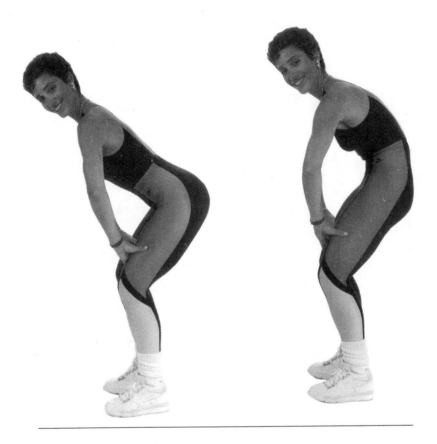

1.

Stand with your feet hip width apart. Put your hands on your thighs; your knees are soft and back is flat. Inhale.

2.

Exhale. Round the upper and lower back in four counts. Hold for eight counts.

3.

Return to beginning position in four counts.

4.

Repeat four times.

6. Reaches

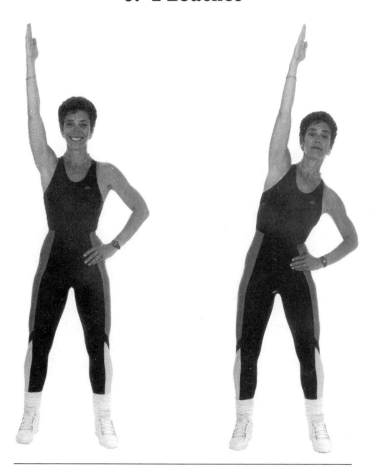

1.

Stand with your feet hip width apart. Put one hand on your hip and one arm straight up in the air with the palm facing your head. The shoulders press down; knees are soft; abs are in.

2.

Reach and stretch to the side for two counts. Return to center. Repeat eight times.

3.

Repeat to the other side.

4.

Hold position 2 for eight counts. Hold position 3 for eight counts.

7. Tricep Squat

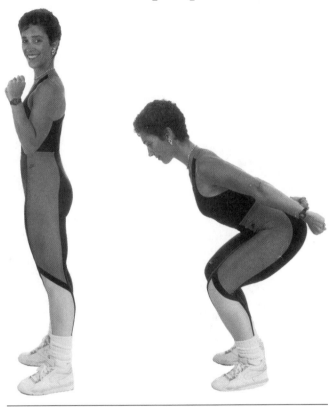

1.

Stand with your feet hip distance apart with the knees soft. Your arms should be bent with the thumbs toward the face. Inhale.

2.

Exhale. Squat back as if you are sitting in a chair. Knees are midway over the arch of the foot with the weight into your heels. Your back is at an angle, chest is up; arms then straighten (tricep extension). Elbows are higher than your back. Perform in four counts.

3.

Return to beginning position in four counts.

4.

Repeat eight times.

8. Deltoid (Shoulder) Lunges

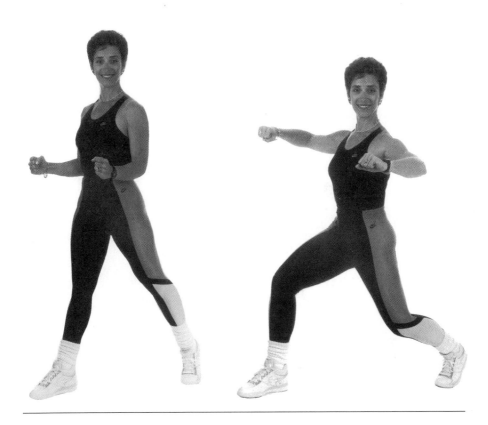

1.

Stand with one foot forward. The other foot is back and the toe is up. The weight is on the forward foot. Arms are bent at ninety degrees. The thumbs are up. Inhale.

2.

Exhale. Drop the torso down by bending the knee. Keep the buttocks higher than the knees. Press down into the front heel. Raise the arms up to the side to shoulder height. Perform in four counts. Return to beginning position in four counts.

3.

Repeat on the other leg.

4.

Repeat eight times for each leg.

9. Shoulder Extensions

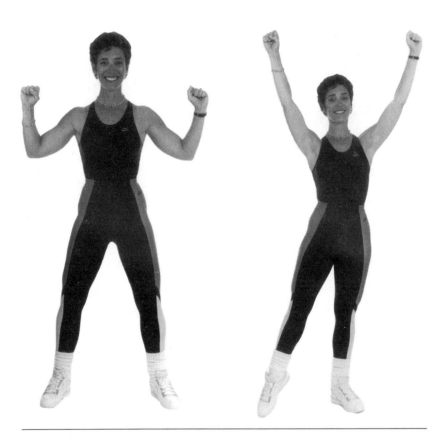

1.

Stand with your feet hip distance apart. Arms are bent at the elbow, midway to the waist. Knees are soft, abs in. Inhale.

2.

Exhale. Extend the arms. Push your weight over to one leg and point the toe of the opposite foot.

3.

Return directly to the other leg.

4.

Repeat sixteen times.

10. Chest Presses

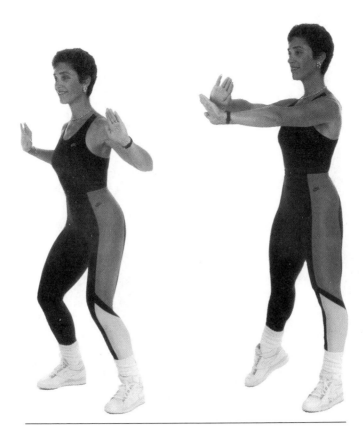

1.

Stand with your feet hip distance apart. Knees are soft, abs in. Pull elbows back and stretch your chest.

2.

Push palms forward; cross the right hand over the left hand, keeping the back straight. Squeeze the chest; point the right toe.

3.

Cross the left hand over the right hand; point the left toe and repeat the exercise on this side.

4.

Repeat for sixteen counts.

11. Lat Pulldowns/Ham Curls

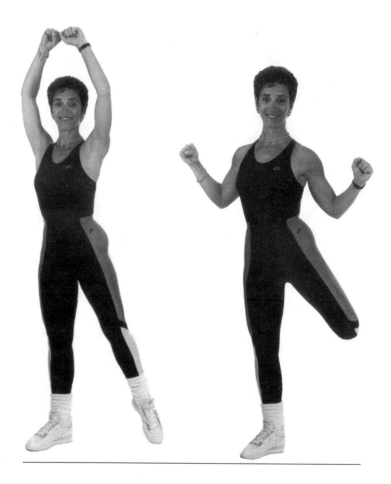

1.

Begin with weight on one leg. Point the other foot. Reach your arms up over your head. Inhale.

2.

Exhale. Pull arms down as your heel lifts back toward your buttocks.

3.

Go directly through the beginning position to the other side.

4.

Repeat sixteen times. Continue to Low Pulls/ Ham Curl.

12. **L**ow Pulls/Ham Curl

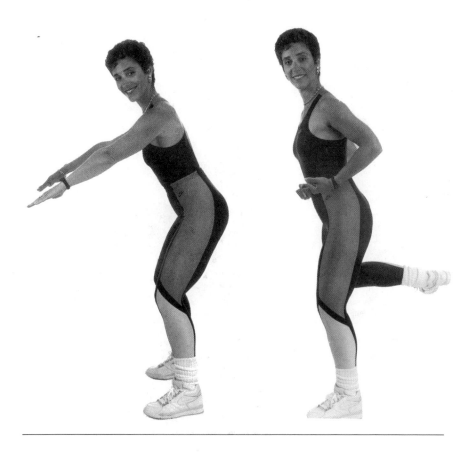

1.

Arms reach forward with the palms down in midway position. Inhale.

2.

Exhale. Pull the arms back, palms up, as heel lifts back. Continue right on to other side.

3.

Repeat sixteen times.

13. Bicep Curl/Knee Lift

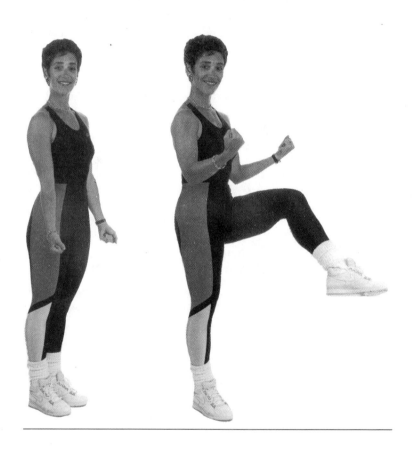

1.

Stand with your feet together. Pull abs in; knees are soft. Keep your body lifted. Inhale.

2.

Exhale. Lift one knee and pull hands toward shoulders, keeping elbows still.

3.

Continue same arm movement with other leg.

4.

Repeat sixteen times.

STRETCHING

Stretching is a vital part of the warm-up. As we get older we lose our flexibility, which increases the risk of injury. Stretching muscles gives them a greater range of motion. Proper stretching allows our muscles to become more flexible and cuts down on injury.

In Molly Fox's Step On It program you will stretch before and after the cardiovascular exercises. The stretches at the end of the workout should be held for twenty to thirty seconds for the maximum benefit. Stretch to the point of gentle release; never stretch through pain. Remember to relax and don't bounce. Breathe deeply as you stretch and exhale fully. Stretching feels good—enjoy it.

14. Shoulder Stretch

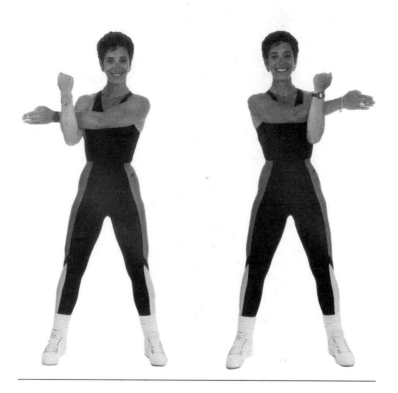

1.

Stand with your feet hip distance apart. Cross one arm over your chest. Hold in place with the other arm for sixteen counts.

2.

Repeat with the other arm.

Keep the back wide, chest lifted, and shoulders pressed down.

15. **H**ip Flexor

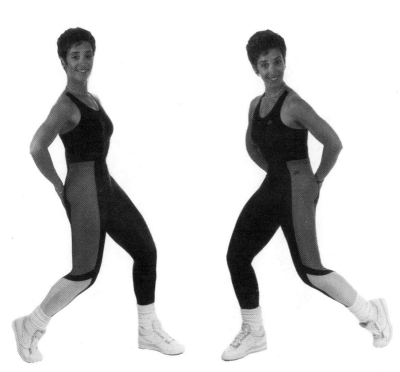

1.

Stand with one foot forward. The other foot is back and on the toe. The weight is on the forward foot. Place your hands on the buttocks. Inhale. Exhale and squeeze buttocks into a pelvic tilt, holding the abs in tightly. The thigh should be pressed slightly back. You should feel the stretch where your leg meets your torso. Hold for sixteen counts.

2.

Repeat on the other side.

16. Quadricep Stretch

1.

Balance on your left leg. Bring the right foot back by holding onto the foot with the right hand from the outside. Reach the left arm up; keep thumbs back. Add a slight pelvic tilt. Keep abs pulled in. To release the pressure from the knee, gently push the foot into the hand. Hold for sixteen counts.

2.

Repeat with the left leg.

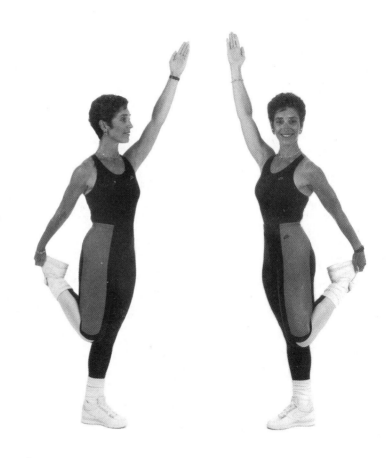

17. **H**amstring Stretch

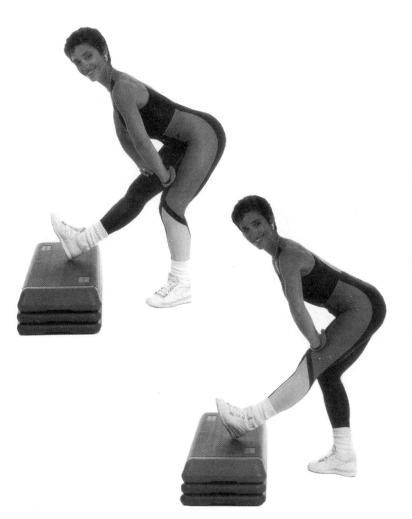

1.

Extend your right leg forward onto the step. Flex your heel, and keeping weight back on the left foot, slightly bend the left knee. Place the hands on the thighs. Make sure the back is long and flat. Abs should be pulled in; neck should be long. Hold this for sixteen counts. Feel the back of the right leg stretch.

2.

Repeat on the other leg.

18. Inner Thigh Stretch

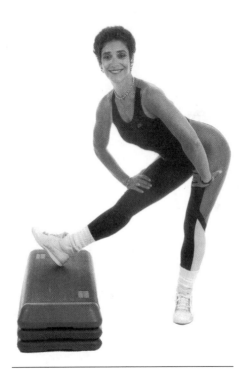

1.

Extend your right leg forward onto the step. Turn the left leg so that the foot and knee face to the left. This will stretch the inner part of the right leg. Hold for sixteen counts.

2.

Repeat with the left leg.

19. Calf Warm-up

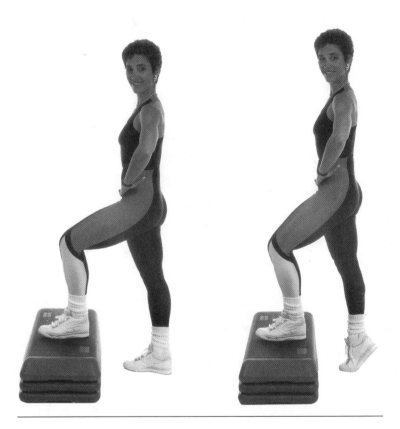

1.

Place the left foot on the step. Place your hands on your hips. Your weight should be back on the right foot.

2.

Rise onto the right toe by lifting your body weight straight up. Then lower the heel to the floor. Repeat eight times.

3.

Repeat with the other leg.

20. More Calf Warm-up

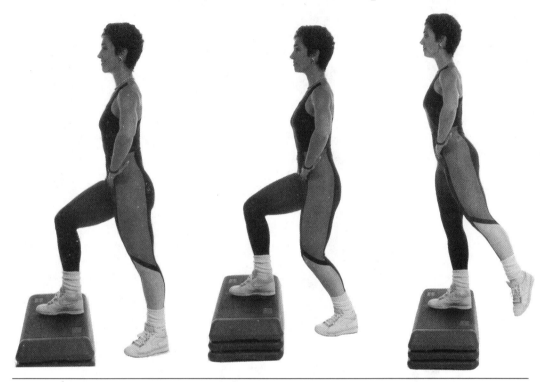

1.

Place right leg on the step. Bend the left knee. Keep the heel down. Then push the whole body weight up onto the right foot. Your left foot will be stretched back. Drop left foot to the floor in a toe-ball-heel motion. Repeat eight times. Then hold left foot on the floor with the knee bent for sixteen counts.

2.

Repeat with the left leg.

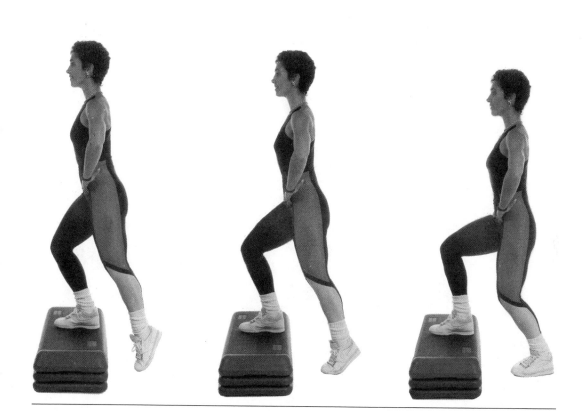

21. Calf Stretches

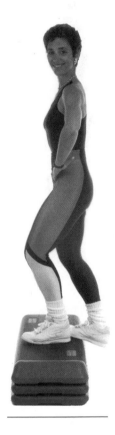

1.

Place both feet on the step. Drop the right heel off the edge of the step. Keep legs straight and the body lifted. Do not force the stretch. Hold for sixteen counts.

2.

Repeat with the left heel.

CONDITIONING

The conditioning program in *Molly Fox's Step On It* has been designed to strengthen the major muscle groups of the upper and lower body. By performing these exercises you will increase lean muscle mass (body composition) and develop shapely muscles. Muscle conditioning is also very important for preventing injury. The conditioning exercises should be performed three times a week. You should rest one day in between each weight workout.

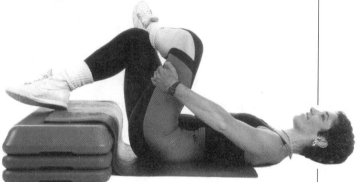

Weights

Weights should only be used when you are sure of your footing. Weights are *not* recommended for anyone who has:

• lower back problems

• high blood pressure

• a history of heart disease

• arthritis

• a significant weight problem

Women who are past the second trimester of pregnancy should also not use weights.

Novices or beginners should not use weights at all. Intermediate steppers may use one- or two-pound weights. Advanced steppers or athletes may use three-pound weights. *Weights are always optional.* You will still get a full workout without using weights.

Any of the conditioning exercises may be performed without using weights. If you *are* using weights, keep checking your form. If you have bad form, use lighter weights or don't use weights at all. If you are a woman and are afraid of developing huge muscles—relax—you have to lift *very* heavy weights over a long period of time to add significant muscle mass. One- to three-pound weights will only *tone* your upper body.

Mats

For your comfort, and a little extra padding, you might want to place a towel or mat (as pictured) on the step while performing the conditioning exercises.

One final note on the conditioning exercises: Any of these exercises may be performed standing up. If you have lower back pain, please do the exercises standing up (instead of sitting on the step).

1. **A**bdominals

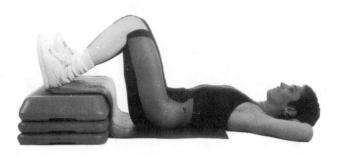

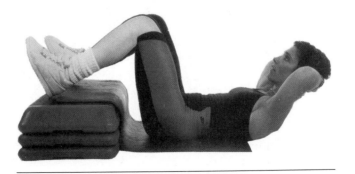

1.

Lie on your back. Rest your heels on top of the step and keep your buttocks close to the step (four to six inches away). Clasp your hands behind your head. Inhale.

2.

Exhale. Lift your upper back for one count.

3.

Lift your right heel; pull your right knee in about four inches; then lift the upper back two more inches.

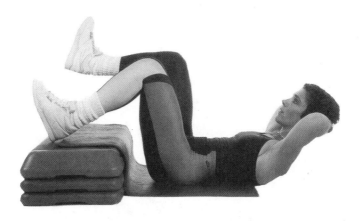

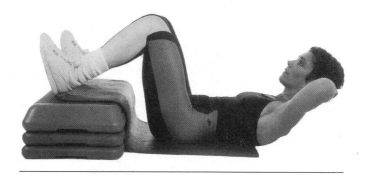

4.

Lower both your heel and upper body until the shoulder blades touch the floor.

5.

Repeat the exercise with the left leg. Alternate each leg sixteen times.

2. Crunches—Holds and Pulses

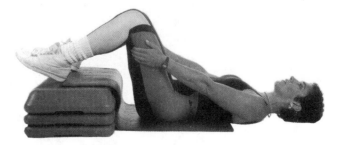

1.

Rest your heels on the step. Reach forward and grab the outside of your thighs. Inhale.

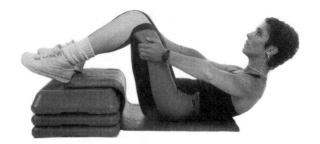

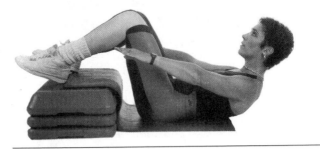

Variation One—for Beginners

Exhale. Curl up. Flex the abdominal muscles. Keep the shoulders up off the floor. Exhale again. Pulse one inch and release. Repeat pulsing one inch and releasing eight times. Then rest back.

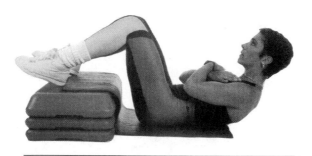

Variation Two—for Beginners

Exhale. Grab the outside of your legs, hold; then place your arms across your chest and pulse one inch and release one inch. Repeat eight times.

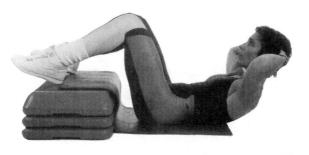

Variation Three—for Intermediate

Exhale. Grab the outside of your legs; hold; then clasp your hands behind your head. Pulse up and down eight times.

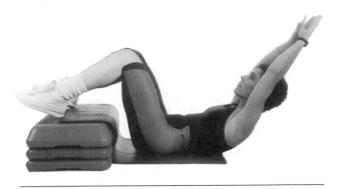

Variation Four—for Advanced

Exhale. Grab the outside of your legs; hold; then bring arms up by your head. Pulse up one inch and down one inch. Repeat eight times.

Perform your variation of choice three to four sets (eight repetitions equals a set).

3. Obliques—Holds and Pulses

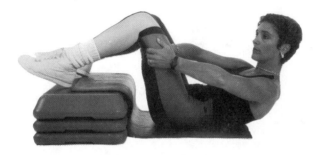

1.

Grab the inside and outside of your left thigh with both hands. Stretch your back and crunch your abdominals. Hold.

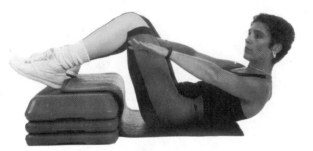

2.

Release your arms; keep the height; push the shoulders down. Pulse eight times.

3.

Variation two.

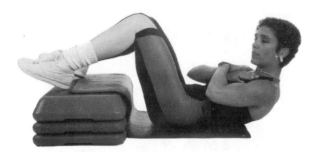

4.

Variation three.

5.

Variation four.

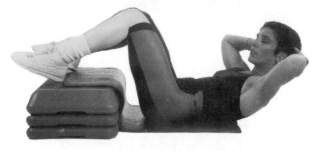

Repeat with the right leg. Do one to four sets of your variation of choice.

4. Center Abdominal Pulses

1.

Rest your heels on the step, hands outstretched between your legs. Inhale.

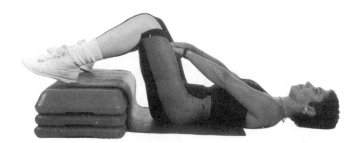

2.

Exhale. Curl up; pulse up and down one inch. Repeat sixteen times.

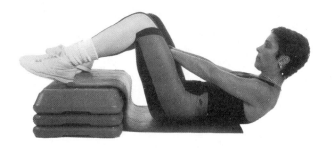

Upper Abdominal Pulses

1.

Start with your heels resting on the step and your hands on your knees. Inhale.

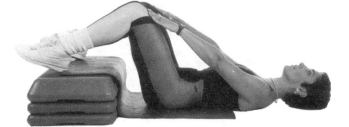

2.

Exhale. Curl up while sliding your hands forward on knees and then down one inch. Repeat sixteen times.

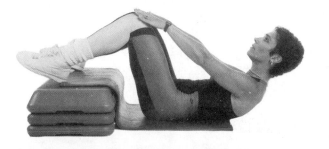

5. Oblique Curls and Pulses

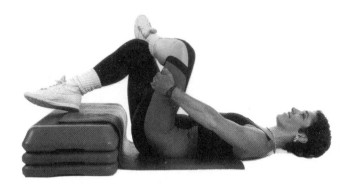

1.

Heels on the step. Cross your left leg over your right leg. Reach your left arm to left leg. Right hand is behind your head.

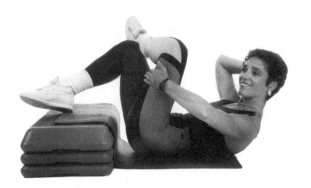

2.

Curl up until shoulder blades come off the floor then curl back until shoulder blades touch. Repeat eight times.

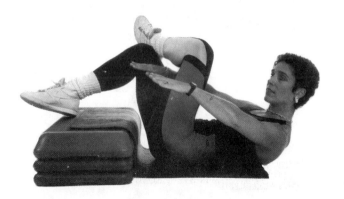

3.

Reach both arms forward and pulse. Press shoulders down. Repeat eight to sixteen times. Reach rib cage to the hipbone.

6. Chest and Triceps—Incline Push-ups

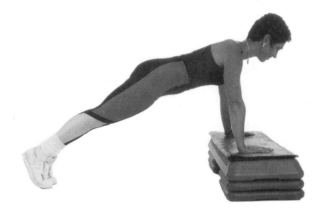

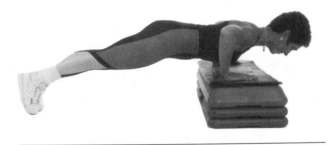

1.

Put your hands on the step. Chest lines up with the heels of your hands.

2.

Pitch your weight slightly forward; drop your chest to the step by bending the elbows. Inhale. Keep abs in tight, legs strong, and butt squeezed.

3.

Exhale. Push up to beginning position— straight arms.

4.

Repeat ten to thirty times.

Beginners should modify this exercise by pushing up from a knee position (get on knees, cross the feet at the angle, pitch forward, and follow the rest of the exercise) until they get stronger.

7. **T**ricep Dips

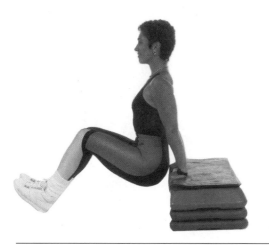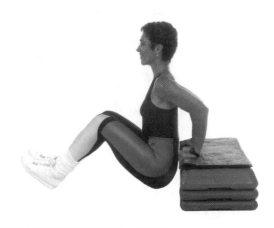

1.

Put your back toward the step; keep heels on the floor. Put the heels of your hands on the edge of the step; line up the shoulders and the hips. Roll the shoulders slightly forward. Inhale.

2.

Bend elbows; drop hips to floor, shoulders down.

3.

Exhale. Straighten arms and push up. Keep shoulders pressed down throughout the exercise.

4.

Repeat ten to thirty times.

8. **B**ench Presses (use heavier weights)

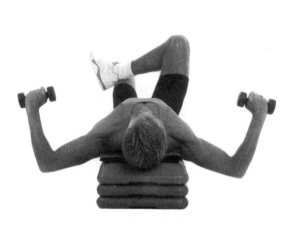 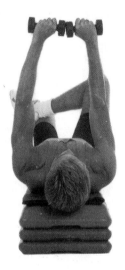

1.

Lie on the step; keep one foot on the floor, and cross the other leg over. Keep your back flat on the step. Drop the elbows toward the floor, stretching the chest. Inhale.

2.

Exhale. Extend arms straight up and through the weights. Arms must stay lined up with the chest muscles. Keep abdominals pulled in.

3.

Repeat twelve to twenty times for one to three sets.

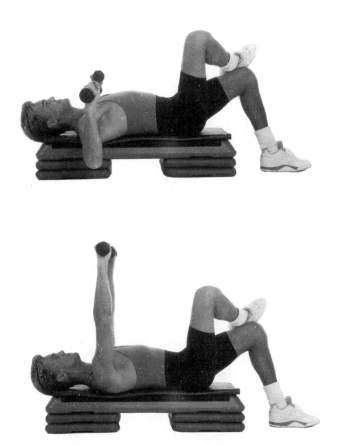

9. Chest Flys (use medium weights)

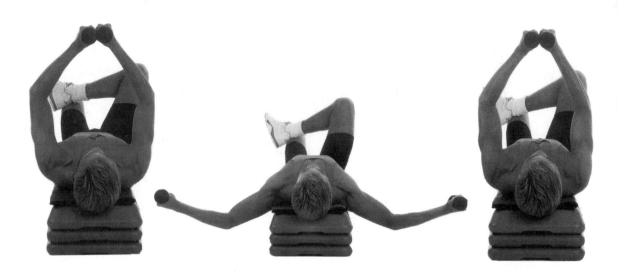

1.
Lie on the step; keep one foot on the floor and cross the other leg over. Begin with your arms rounded (pretend that you are holding a beach ball); shoulders press down; back is into the step; abs are pulled in.

2.
Inhale. Drop the elbows toward the floor, keeping the shoulders pressed down. You should feel the stretch in the chest and the front of the shoulder muscles.

3.
Exhale. Bring the hands back to the original position.

4.
Repeat twelve to twenty times for one to three sets.

You must keep your back flat on the step at all times.

10. Pullovers—Chest and Triceps
(use light to medium weights)

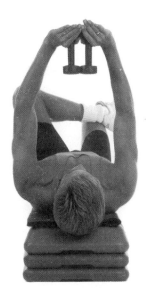 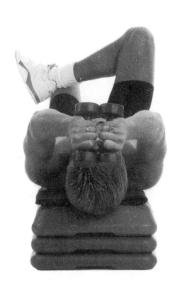 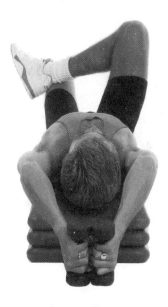

1.
Lie on the step; keeping one foot on the floor, cross the other leg over. Begin with weights held between the thumb and index finger.

2.
Inhale. Stretch your arms back from the shoulder, keeping them slightly bent. You should feel a stretch in the triceps around the rib cage and back. Keep your back down.

3.
Carefully lower your arms to the floor. Exhale. Pull over your chest and back to the original position. You should feel a pull down in your rib cage.

4.
Repeat twelve to twenty times for one to three sets.

11. Tricep Extensions
(use medium to heavy weights)

1.

Lie on the step, keeping one foot on the floor. Press your shoulders down. Bend your elbows. Touch the weights to your chest. Inhale.

2.

Exhale. Extend elbows. Push weights up to straight position and back to original position.

3.

Repeat twelve to twenty times for one to three sets.

12. **U**pper Tricep Extensions
(use medium weights)

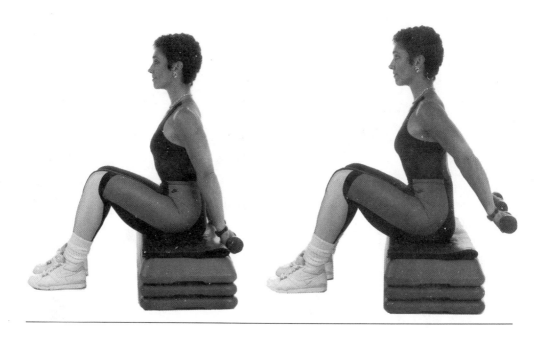

1.

Sit up on the step with buttocks at the back end of the step. Start with your arms back on either side of your hips, behind the step. Inhale.

2.

Exhale. Lift straight arms back and squeeze the upper triceps and shoulders.

3.

Return to the original position.

4.

Repeat twelve to twenty times for one to three sets.

13. Traditional Tricep Extensions (use medium weights)

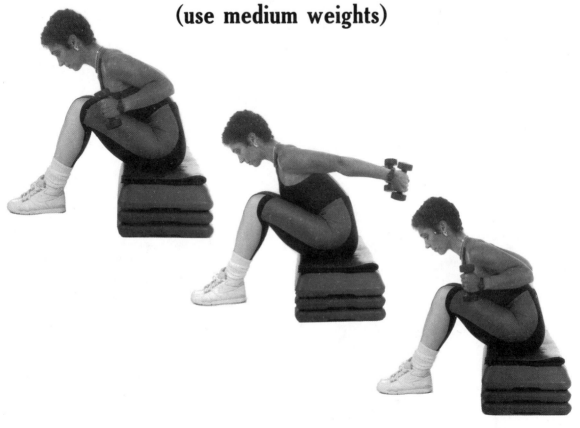

1.
Sit up on the step with buttocks at the back end of the step. Bend over; try to rest your chest on your legs; bring weights in toward shoulders, keeping elbows high. Inhale.

2.
Exhale. Extend arms back, tighten the triceps, and squeeze.

3.
Return to the original position.

4.
Repeat twelve to twenty times for one to three sets.

14. Back and Biceps—Lat Rows (use heavy weights)

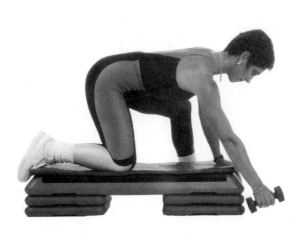 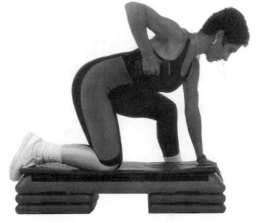

1.

Put your right knee on the step, left foot just next to the step, left hand on the edge of the step. Drop your right arm down and forward, feeling a stretch in the outer back muscles. Inhale.

2.

Exhale. Pull the weight back, keeping the elbow high and the shoulder down. You should feel a squeeze in the outer back muscle.

3.

Repeat on other side.

4.

Repeat twelve to twenty times for one to three sets.

15. Upright Rows
(use medium weights)

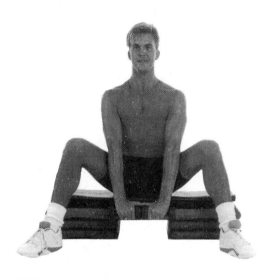 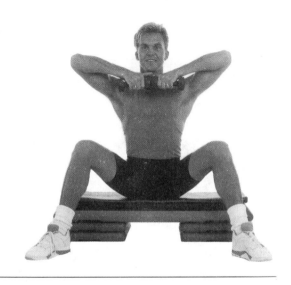

1.

Sit on the step. Keep your back lifted up, abs in, feet wide. Arms are extended down; weights are together. You should feel a slight squeeze in the chest. Inhale.

2.

Exhale. Pull the weights up under your chin; keep them close to the body, elbows high and shoulders down.

3.

Lower to original position.

4.

Repeat twelve to twenty times for one to three sets.

16. Bent-over Wide Rows
(use medium weights)

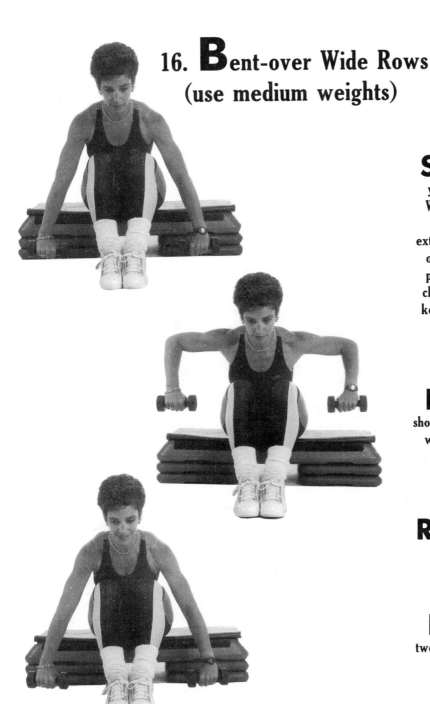

1.

Sit on the step with your feet together. Weights are in both hands; arms are extended near the heel of the foot; abs are pulled in. Rest your chest on your thighs; keep your neck long. Inhale.

2.

Exhale. Keep your shoulders down; pull the weights up; squeeze back muscles.

3.

Return to the original position.

4.

Repeat twelve to twenty times for one to three sets.

17. Erector Spinal and Glutes

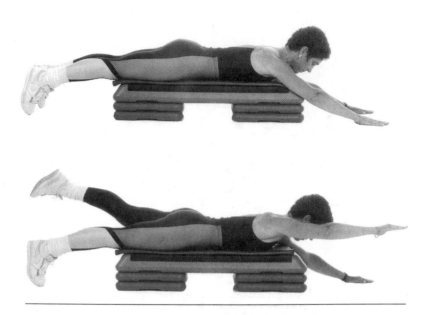

1.

Lie with your stomach on the step, toes touching the floor. Extend your arms out in front of you with both hands on the floor. Keep your abs in; stretch your neck long. Inhale.

2.

Exhale. Lift the right arm and left leg in four counts. Lower for four counts.

3.

Repeat the exercise with the left arm and right leg.

4.

Alternate sides for twelve to twenty repetitions.

18. Upper Back
(use light weights)

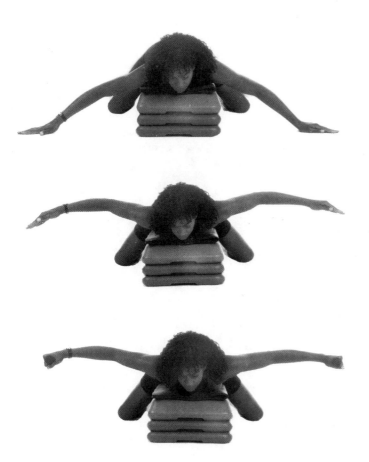

1.

Lie with your stomach on the step; drop your knees to the floor, and relax. Put arms out to the side, keep your neck long and palms on the floor. Rotate armpits down. Inhale.

2.

Exhale. Lift arms up and squeeze shoulder blades together for four counts. Then lower for four counts.

3.

Repeat twelve to twenty times.

19. Bicep Curls
(use medium to heavy weights)

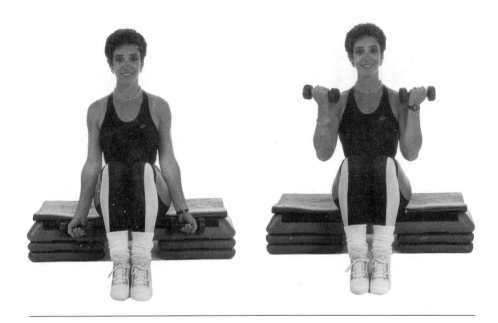

1.

Sit on the step; keep your feet together, abs pulled in, back and chest up straight, arms at your sides, palms facing forward. Inhale.

2.

Exhale. Curl weights up to your shoulder, squeeze biceps, and return to beginning position.

3.

Repeat twelve to twenty times for one to three sets.

20. Bottom Half/Top Half

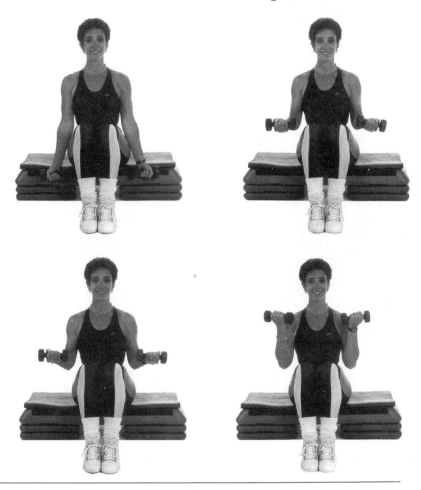

1.

Sit on the step; keep your feet together, abs pulled in, back and chest up straight, arms at your sides, palms facing forward. Inhale.

2.

Curl halfway up; lower all the way down; squeeze biceps. Repeat twelve to twenty times.

3.

Start halfway up, then curl all the way up, lower halfway down, squeeze biceps. Repeat twelve to twenty times.

21. Hammer Curls
(use medium to heavy weights)

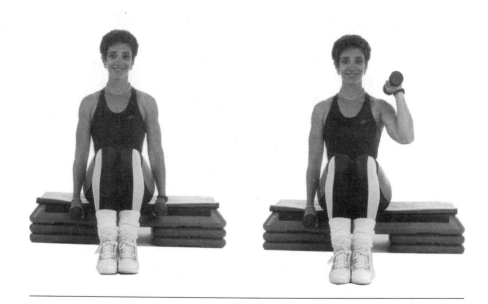

1.

Sit on the step; keep your feet together, abs pulled in, back and chest up straight, arms at your sides, palms facing in toward each other.

2.

Curl left weight toward the shoulder; switch right weight toward shoulder. Keep alternating from right to left for twelve to twenty repetitions, one to three sets.

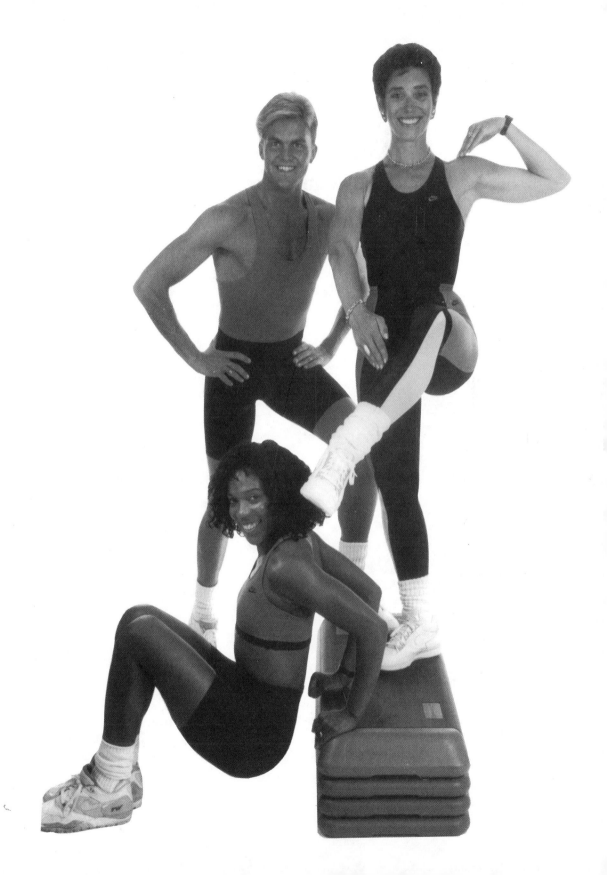

22. Bicep and Shoulder combo
(use medium to heavy weights)

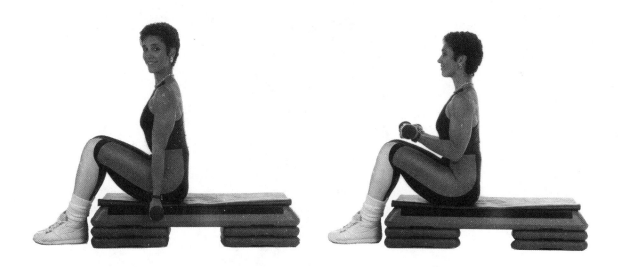

1.
Sit on the front or end of the step with your arms down and abs in.

2.
Curl weights to your shoulder, keeping palms toward the shoulder.

3.
Rotate wrists so that palms are facing out, and push weights straight overhead, shoulders down.

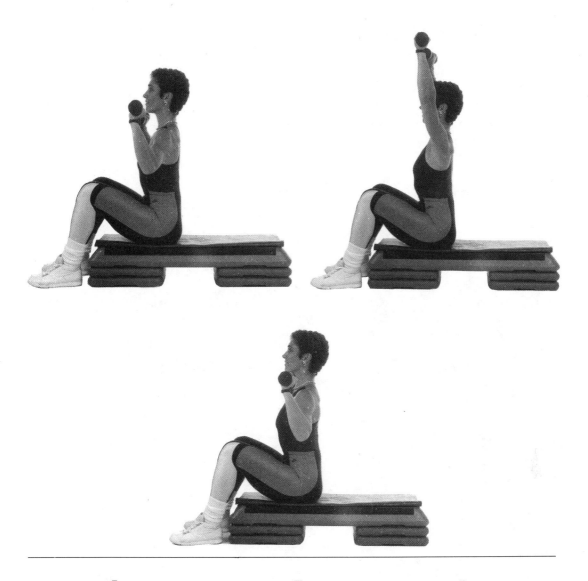

4.

Lower weights to shoulders.

5.

Rotate palms; extend arms down to original position.

6.

Repeat twelve to twenty times for one to three sets.

23. Round the World Shoulder
(use medium weights)

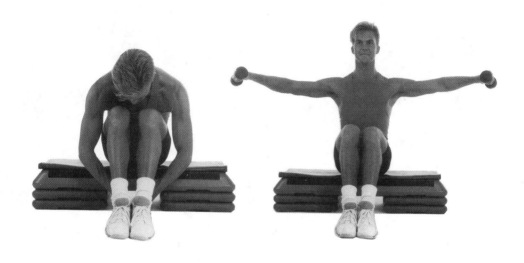

1.

Sit on the step; rest your chest on your thighs; keep your shoulders down and your arms rounded with weights touching under the legs. Inhale.

2.

Exhale. Arms come out to the side at shoulder height.

3.

Arms come together overhead with hands slightly in front of the shoulders; keep the elbows bent and the shoulders down. Inhale.

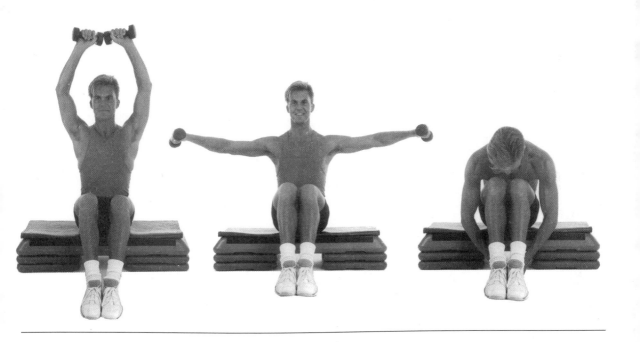

4.

Exhale. Stretch arms out and down, palms to floor at shoulder height.

5.

Return to original position.

6.

Repeat twelve to twenty times for one to three sets.

24. Shoulder Pulses (use medium weights)

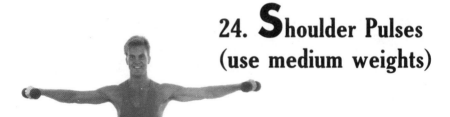

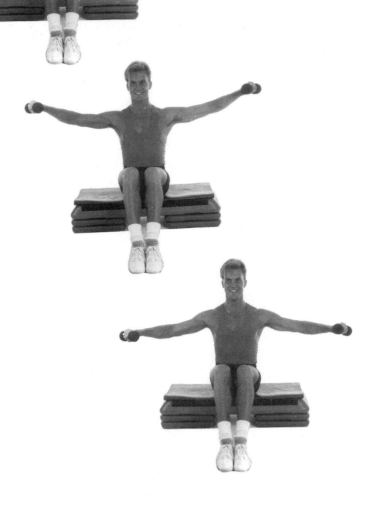

1.

Sit on the step; stretch arms out to the side at shoulder height.

2.

Lift arms up three inches and down three inches (so that hands are below the shoulders). Make sure to keep your back straight, abs in, and throat and neck soft.

3.

Do twelve to twenty repetitions.

25. **R**ear Delts
(use medium weights)

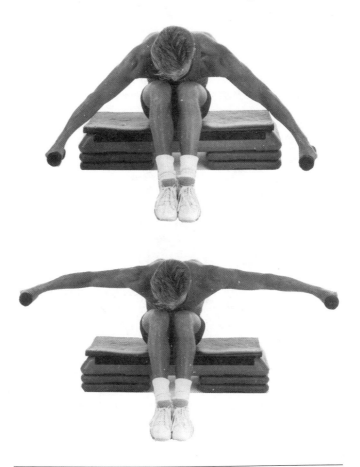

1.

Sit on the step; rest the chest on the thighs; put arms under the legs. Inhale.

2.

Exhale. Extend arms out and up to shoulder height. Keep shoulders down; squeeze the shoulder blades.

3.

Repeat twelve to twenty times for one to three sets.

26. Shoulder Presses
(use medium weights)

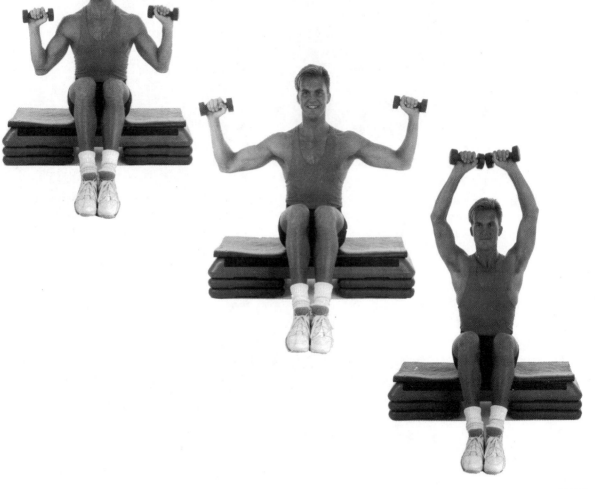

1.

Sit on the step; keep your back up, abs in, and shoulders down.

2.

Push weights up; keep shoulders down to midway position.

3.

Touch weights at the top over your head for four counts each way.

4.

Repeat twelve to twenty times for one to three sets.

27. Single Front Shoulder Raises
(use medium weights)

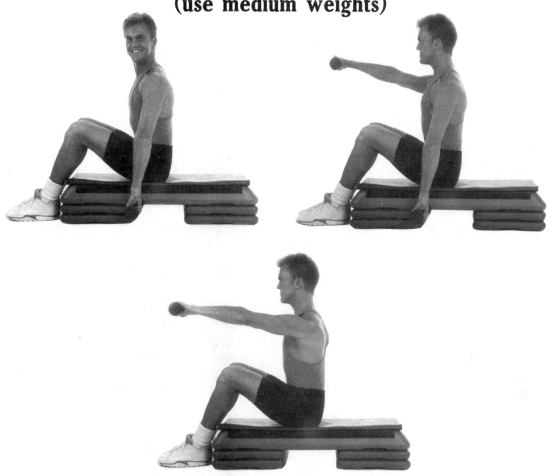

1.

Sit on the end or front of the step.

2.

Raise your right arm up to shoulder height. Be sure to keep your shoulders down and your back up.

3.

Lower arm down to beginning and then lift left arm and return to beginning position. Four counts each way.

4.

Repeat twelve to twenty times for one set only.

28. Double Front Raises

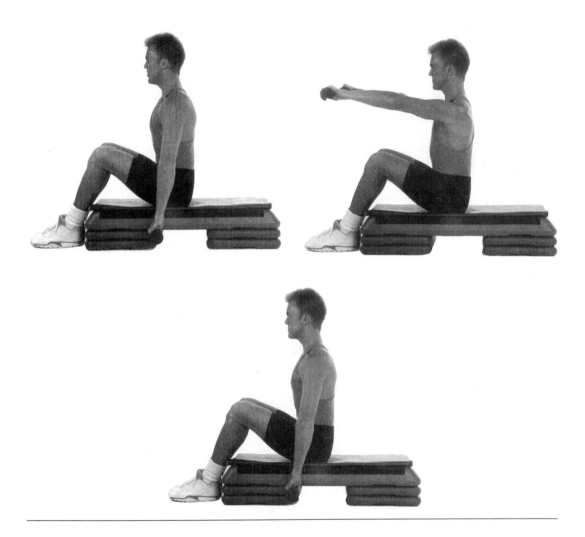

1.
Sit on the end or front of the step.

2.
Raise both arms up to shoulder height. Be sure to keep your shoulders down and your back up.

3.
Lower arms down to the beginning position. Four counts each way. Repeat twelve times.

Legs

29. Hip Lifts
(use one to two pound leg weights—optional)

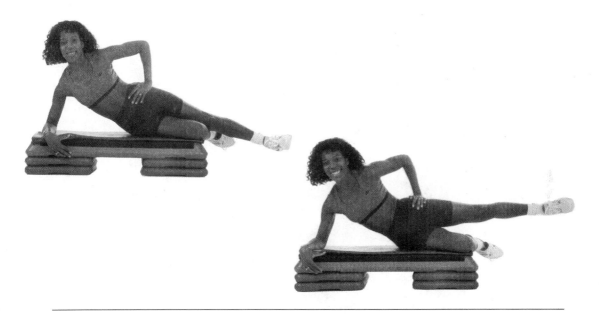

1.

Lie on the step. Come up on one elbow; keep stomach and ribs pulled in, shoulders down. You should feel your weight press into the bottom leg, which is bent. Extend top leg.

2.

Lift your leg up to your hip for four counts. This is a very small motion. Then lower it for four counts until you are in the original position.

3.

Repeat twelve to twenty times for three sets.

Make sure that your top hip does not lift up. Hold your hand on your hip to keep it in place.

30. Rear Leg Extensions

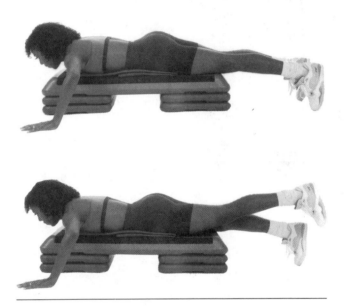

1.

Lie on the step, facedown, hands on the floor, abs in, toes on the floor.

2.

Lift the left leg straight up, four to six inches; four counts up and four counts down. Make sure to squeeze the buttocks as each leg lifts.

3.

Repeat twelve to twenty times for one to three sets on each leg.

If you feel pressure in your lower back put your hands or a towel under your hipbones.

31. **Q**uad and Hip Flexion

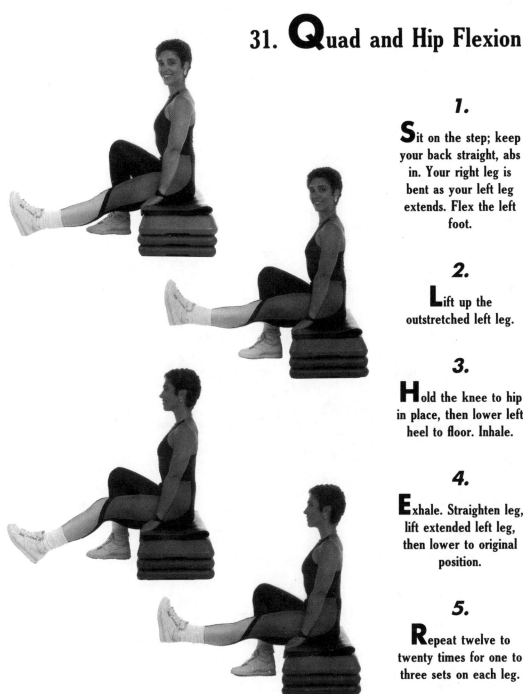

1.

Sit on the step; keep your back straight, abs in. Your right leg is bent as your left leg extends. Flex the left foot.

2.

Lift up the outstretched left leg.

3.

Hold the knee to hip in place, then lower left heel to floor. Inhale.

4.

Exhale. Straighten leg, lift extended left leg, then lower to original position.

5.

Repeat twelve to twenty times for one to three sets on each leg.

32. Quadricep (front of the thigh) Stretch

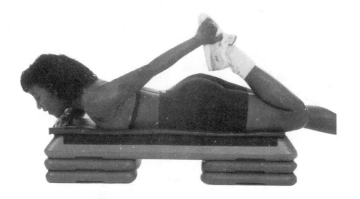

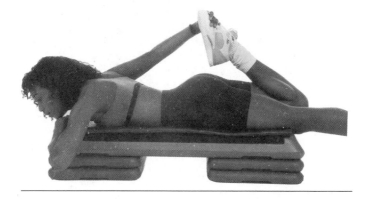

1.

Lie on the step facedown. Grab your left foot from the outside; push your foot into your hand (this will take stress off the knee).

2.

Hold for thirty seconds. Repeat with right foot.

33. Lower Back Stretch

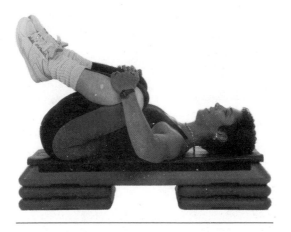

1.

Lie on your back on the step. Pull both knees in toward your chest.

2.

Relax and hold for thirty seconds.

34. Hip Flexor (where the leg meets the pelvis), Hamstring (back of the thigh), and Calf Stretch

1.

Place your buttocks at the end of the step. Extend one leg down to the floor. Pull the other knee in. You can increase the hip flexor stretch by adding a slight pelvic tilt (pulling the pubic bone toward the navel and pulling the abs in). Hold for thirty seconds.

2.

Extend the bent knee. Hold for thirty seconds.

3.

An added bonus—if you flex your foot you will get a good calf stretch.

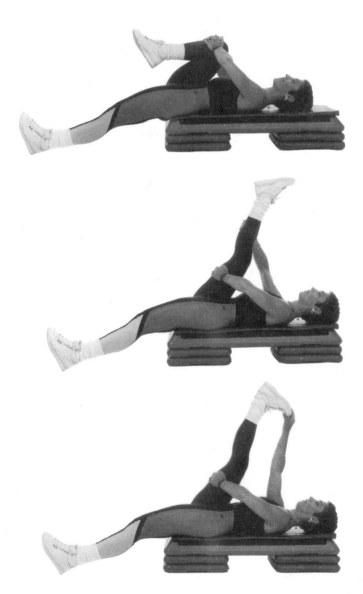

CARDIO WORKOUT

After the stretches and the warm-up it's time to Step On It. Twenty to forty minutes of the cardio section of Molly Fox's Step On It program will reduce body fat, increase lean muscle mass, tone the muscles, and increase cardiorespiratory capacity. Remember to check your pulse after the cardio workout and compare it to the target heart rate chart. Just a reminder—if your heart rate is too high, drop the weights or lower the step height.

The basic cadence for Step On It exercises is *up, up, down, down* (four counts). This sequence is appropriate for all the exercises that lead with the same foot (i.e., right foot steps up, left foot steps up; right foot steps down, left foot steps down). The basic cadence for alternating steps is *up, up, down, tap* (no weight); *up, up, down, down* (i.e., right foot steps up, left foot steps up, right foot steps down, left foot taps down; left foot steps up, right foot steps up, left foot steps down, right foot steps down). The ideal music for Step On It exercises is 120 beats per minute (i.e., Madonna's "Vogue").

Arms and Step On It

Most arm variations can be applied to just about any step exercise. Try experimenting to feel which movements you like best. Always keep your arms down in the low range (waist level) for 60 percent of the stepping time. The arms should be in the mid range (above the waist) or upper range (above the shoulders) for the other 40 percent. If you don't want to use your arms at all, simply keep them loose or on your hips. You will still get an excellent lower body workout. Your arms should stay on your hips until you master the leg movements. Never fling your arms. Always control your movements.

Other Cardio Tips

- If you feel disoriented on the step (everyone will at one time or another), get off and march in place.

- Be sure to fully execute each step. Really climb up on the step using the *thighs* and the *buttocks*.

- The heart rate increase is caused by using the large muscle groups (the large muscles are those in the legs) so keep the legs going even if you stop performing the arm movements.

- To increase the intensity of the workout make your movements *big*.

- Develop a relaxed step cadence. The more relaxed you are the better the workout.

- On *repeaters*—only the toes touch back (no heels, no weight).

- If you experience lower back discomfort, check to be sure that you are not leaning too far over. Stand straight up and lean forward with your entire body (full body lean).

- If your neck feels tight while stepping, soften your arms and let them swing naturally.

- Very important—when you step down think *toe, ball, heel*. Otherwise you might feel extreme calf tightness the next day.

- All steps can be done in place, off the step, if the stepping motion is too intense for you.

How Many Times Should I Do Each Exercise?

Do each exercise for no more than one minute with the same leg leading. For example, if you are doing the Basic Step with the right foot leading, you should change to the left foot leading after one minute. To make the transition to lead with the other foot, just tap (no weight) on the fourth step. Then step up on the step with the same foot.

You do not have to perform each exercise in this section. Choose several different exercises and combine them for a twenty- to forty-minute workout. Mix and match your exercises. Don't forget to warm up and stretch before you Step On It and cool down after you Step On It.

Now go Step On It!

Final Stretch

1. **S**pinal Twist Stretch

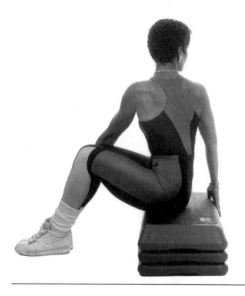 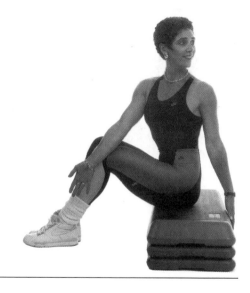

1.

Sit on the step with your knees and feet together. Keep your spine long.

2.

Rotate to the right from the waist. Keep your left arm to the outside of the right thigh and the right arm should be stretched toward the back of the step. Hold for thirty seconds.

3.

Repeat, turning to the left.

Please refer to safety tips on pages 9–18 before beginning these excerises.

2. **T**he Basic Step
(with or without light weights)

1.

Stand with your feet together. Face the step.

2.

Right foot steps up on step.

3.

Left foot steps up on step.

4.

Right foot steps down off step.

5.

Left foot steps down off step.

If you are not using weights keep your hands on your hips.

3. The Basic Step with a Bicep Curl

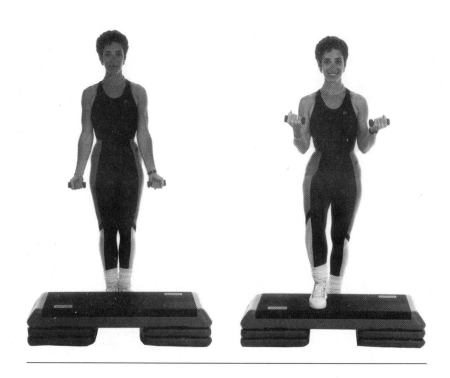

1.

Stand with your feet together, facing step.

2.

Right foot steps up on step, arms curl up.

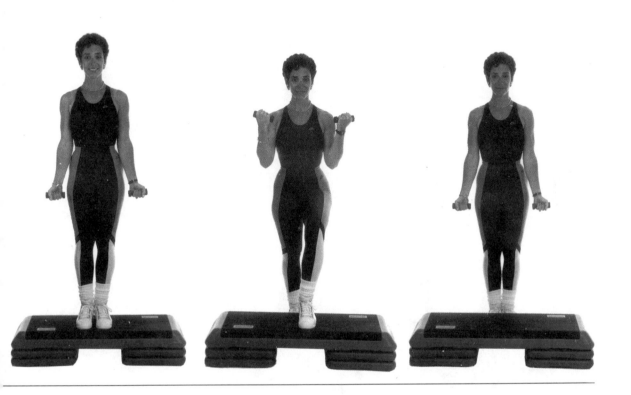

3.

Left foot steps up on step, arms curl down.

4.

Right foot steps down off step, arms curl up.

5.

Left foot steps down off step, arms curl down.

4. The Basic Step with Bicep Curl, Palms Face Up

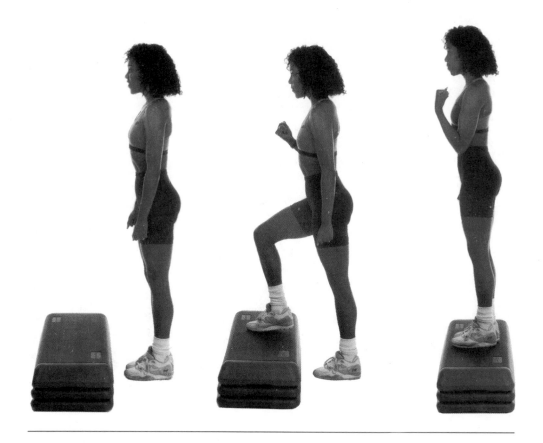

1.

Right foot steps up. Right arm curls up, *palms facing up* toward the shoulders, left arm is down.

2.

Left foot steps up; left arm curls up (both arms are up).

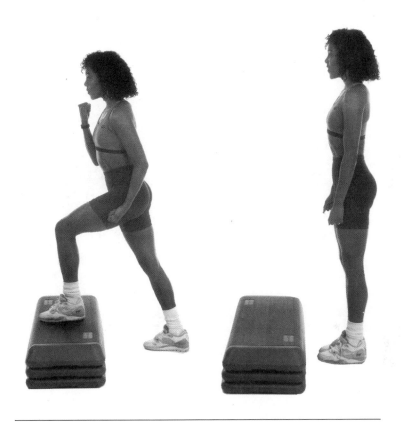

3.

Right foot steps down;
right arm curls down
(left arm is still up).

4.

Left foot steps down;
left arm curls down.

5. The Basic Step with Alternating Hammer Curls, Palms Face Each Other

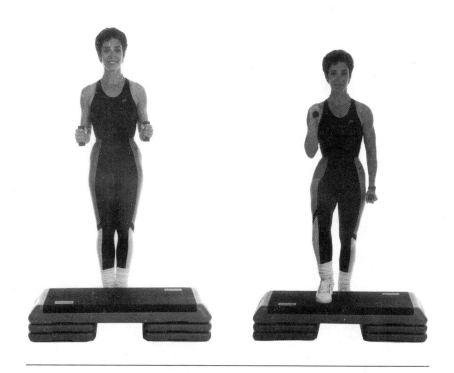

1.

Stand with your feet together, facing the step; both arms are bent at the waist at ninety degrees, palms facing each other.

2.

Right foot steps up. Right arm curls up, *palm facing in*. Left arm is down, palm close to the left outer thigh.

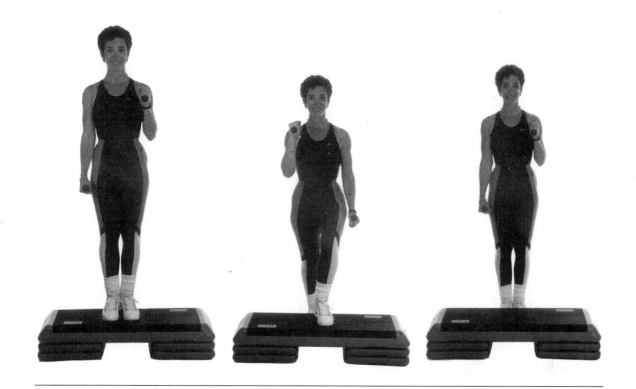

3.

Left foot steps up. Left arm curls up; right arm curls down.

4.

Right foot steps down. Right arm curls up; left arm curls down.

5.

Left foot steps down. Left arm curls up; right arm curls down.

6. The Basic Step with Reverse Bicep Curls

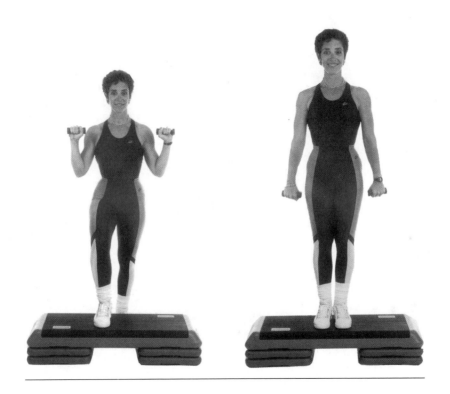

1.

Right foot steps up.
Arms curl up; *knuckles
face up* (the opposite of
a usual bicep position).

2.

Left foot steps up.
Arms curl down;
knuckles face down.

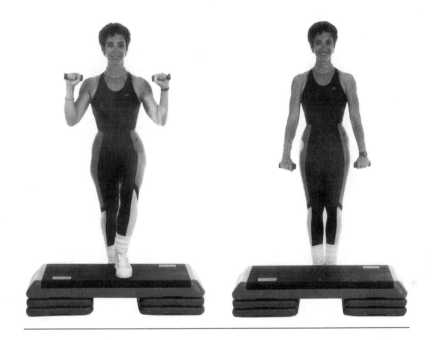

3.

Right foot steps down.
Arms curl up; knuckles
face up.

4.

Left foot steps down.
Arms curl down;
knuckles face down.

7. The Basic Step with Shoulder Rotation

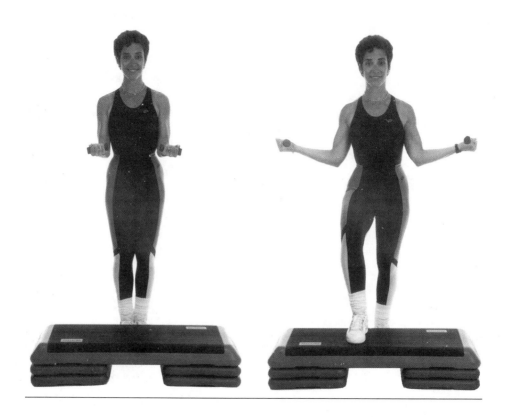

1.

Stand with the legs together; elbows are pinned in at the waist, palms facing up.

2.

As right foot steps up, arms bend at a ninety-degree angle. Hold your elbows still and rotate your shoulders open.

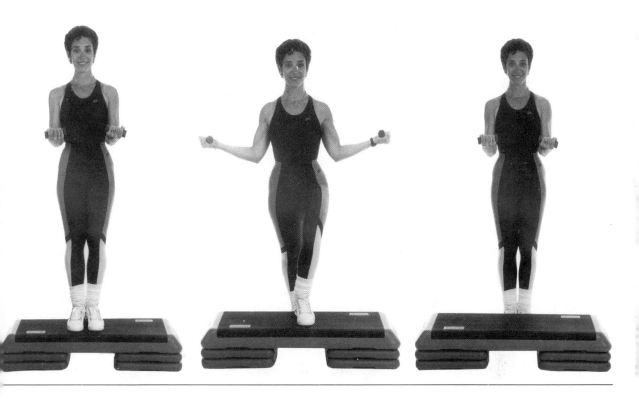

3.

Left foot steps up; shoulders rotate to the beginning position.

4.

Right foot steps down; arms rotate open.

5.

Left foot steps down; arms rotate to the beginning position.

8. The Basic Step with Low Jabs

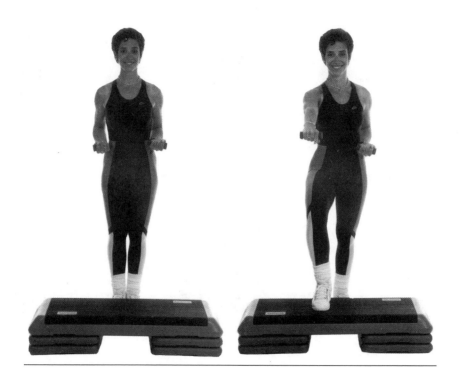

1.

Stand with the legs together; elbows are pinned in at the waist, palms up. Arms are at a ninety-degree angle.

2.

Right foot steps up. Rotate forearm (palm should be down) and extend the right arm forward; left arm remains in place.

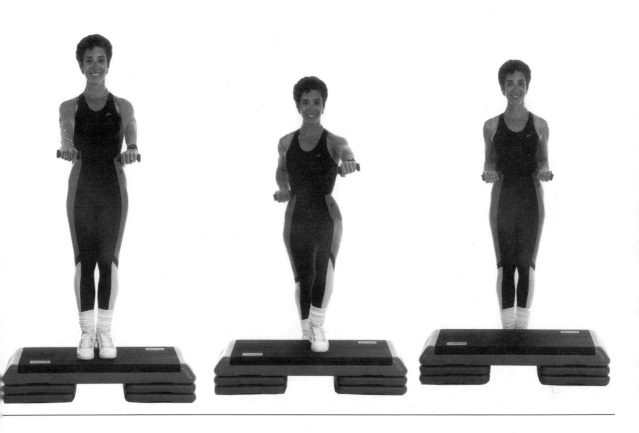

3.

Left foot steps up. Rotate forearm and extend the left arm forward to meet the right arm. The knuckles on both hands are facing up.

4.

Right foot steps down as right arm returns to beginning position (palm is now down again).

5.

Left foot steps down as left arm returns to beginning position.

9. **R**ear Shoulder Lifts/Upper Triceps

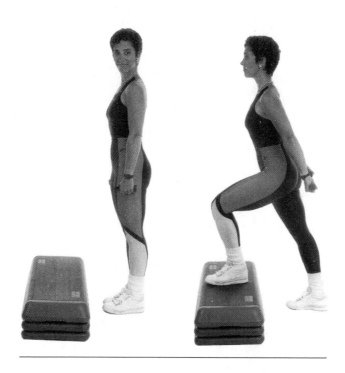

1.
Stand with feet together, arms straight down by your sides.

2.
Left foot steps up. Lift arms up and toward the back; knuckles face your buttocks.

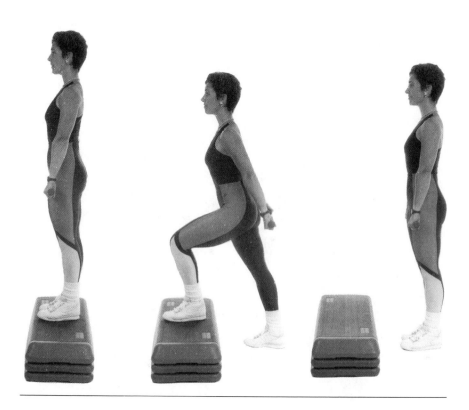

3.

Right foot steps up; lower arms to your side.

4.

Right foot steps down. Lift arms up and toward the back; knuckles face your buttocks.

5.

Left foot steps down; lower arms to your sides.

10. Basic Step with Tricep Extensions

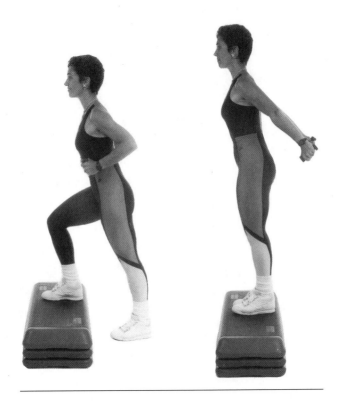

1.

Right foot steps up. Hands are pinned in at the waist; elbows are pointed back and up; hands are in fists.

2.

Left foot steps up. Extend elbows and arms behind the body. Arms are lifted up. (Do not lean forward or arch your back.)

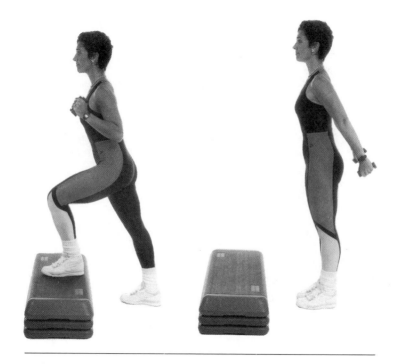

3.

Right foot steps down; curl hands in toward your chest.

4.

Left foot steps down; extend elbows and arms behind the body.

11. Crisscross Basic Step

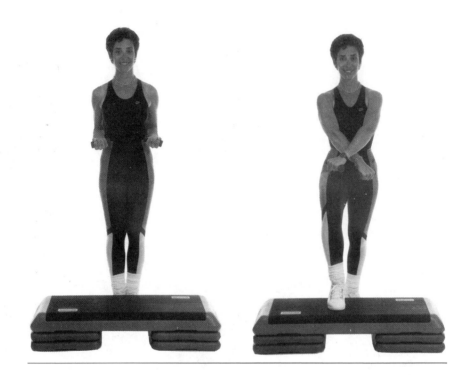

1.

Stand behind the step; arms are bent in ninety-degree angles, palms up.

2.

Right foot steps up; crisscross arms in the front of your body (left arm over the right arm), palms toward the thighs.

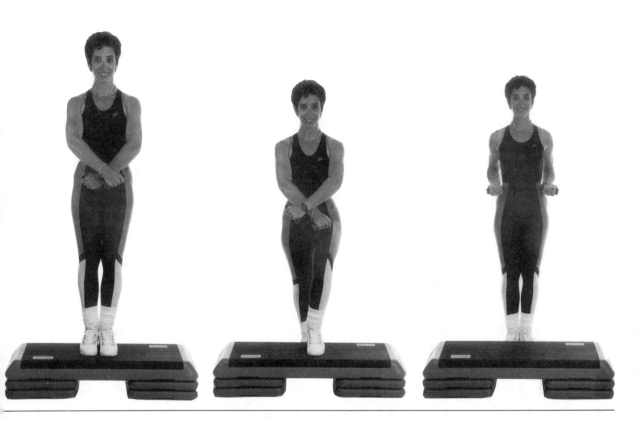

3.
Left foot steps up; cross right arm over left arm in front.

4.
Right foot steps down; cross left arm over right arm in front.

5.
Return to the beginning position.

12. Lateral Shoulder Raises

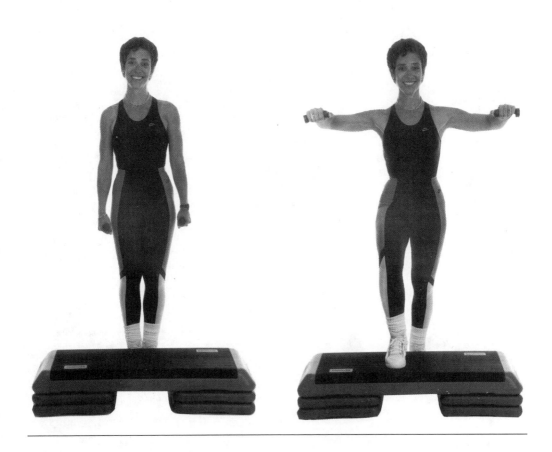

1.

Stand behind the step, arms down by your sides.

2.

Right foot steps up; bend arms at ninety-degree angle, lift to shoulder height.

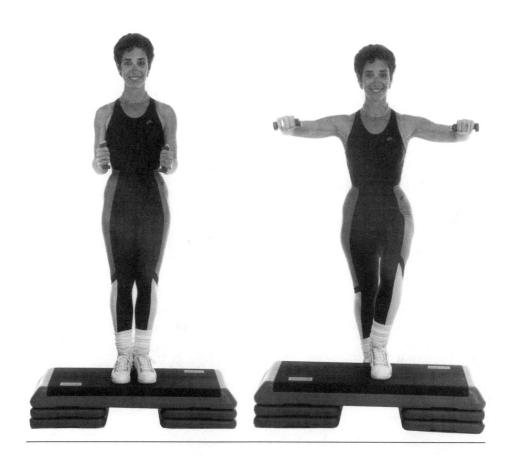

3.

Left foot steps up; lower elbows (elbows are now pinned in at your sides).

4.

Right foot steps down; raise arms to shoulder height.

5.

Left foot steps down; lower elbows and arms back to your sides.

13. Front Shoulder Raises

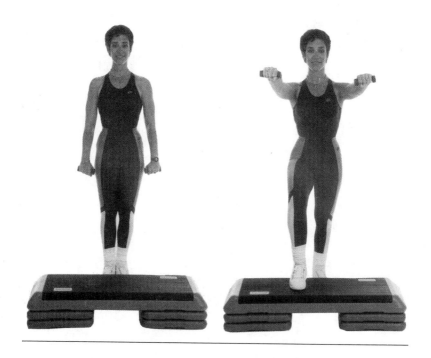

1.
Stand behind the step, arms by your sides, knuckles up.

2.
Right foot steps up; raise both arms straight up to shoulder height. Keep your chest lifted.

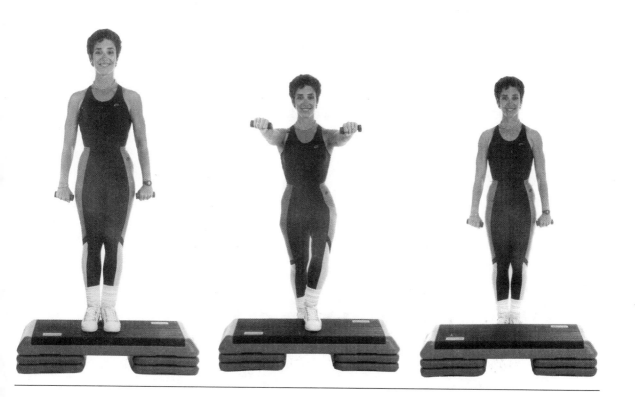

3.

Left foot steps up; both arms lower to your sides.

4.

Right foot steps down; raise both arms straight up to shoulder height.

5.

Left foot steps down; both arms lower to your sides.

14. Mid-Range Bicep Curl

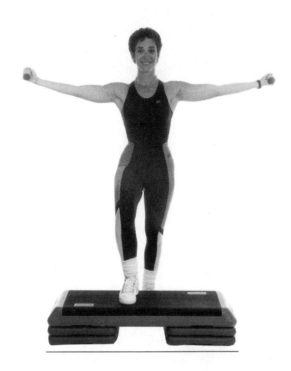

1.
Right foot steps up; arms extended straight out to the side at shoulder height, palms face up.

2.
Left foot steps up; arms curl in; squeeze your biceps.

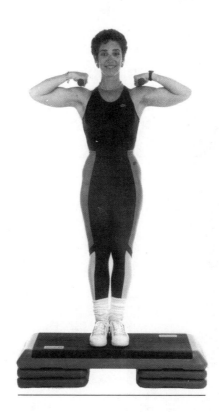

3.

Right foot steps down;
extend arms out to
shoulder height.

4.

Left foot steps down;
arms curl in; squeeze
your biceps.

15. Basic Step with Alternating Mid-Range Bicep Curl

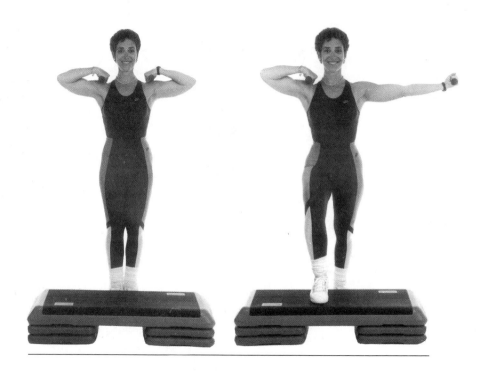

1.

Stand behind the step; arms are curled in at shoulder height, squeezing the bicep, knuckles facing up.

2.

Right foot steps up; extend left arm straight out, palms up. Right arm remains curled in.

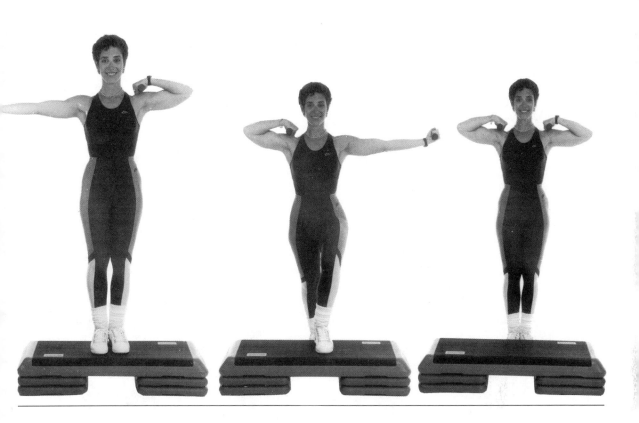

3.

Left foot steps up; alternate arm curls— right arm curls out, left arm curls in.

4.

Right foot steps down; extend left arm straight out, right arm curls in.

5.

Left foot steps down; both arms return to original position.

16. Mid-Range Alternating Under Bicep Curl

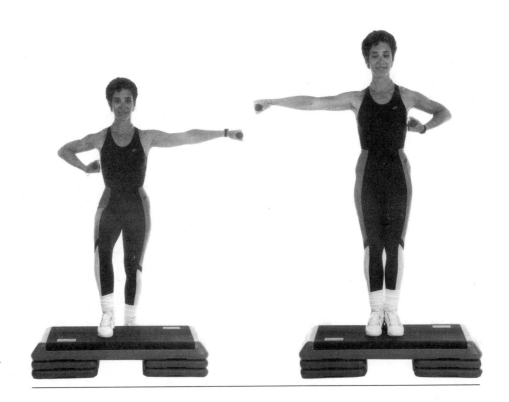

1.

Right foot steps up; curl the right arm under toward the chest, palms facing up; left arm extends straight out to the side.

2.

Left foot steps up; curl the left arm under toward the chest, palm facing up; right arm extends straight out to the side.

Both arms can extend at the same time if desired.

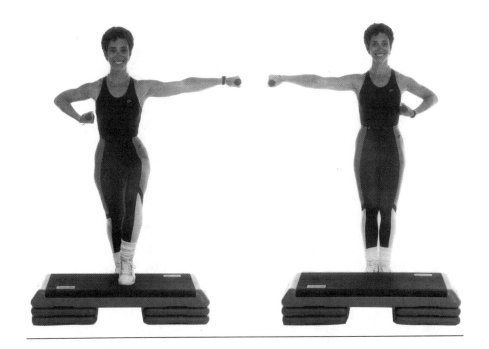

3.

Right foot steps down; curl the right arm under toward the chest, palm facing up; left arm extends straight out to the side.

4.

Left foot steps down; curl the left arm under toward the chest, palm facing up; right arm extends straight out to the side.

17. **M**id-Range Upright Rows

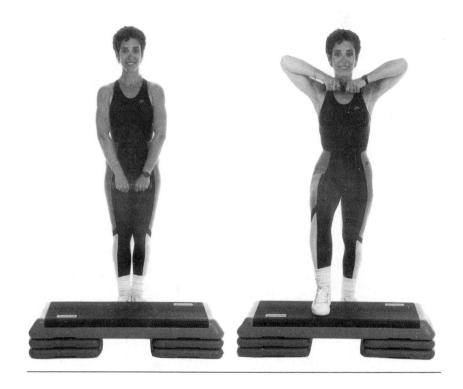

1.

Stand behind the step; arms are down near your thighs, palms facing down.

2.

Right foot steps up; elbows fan out, hands are together; raise the hands up to the chin.

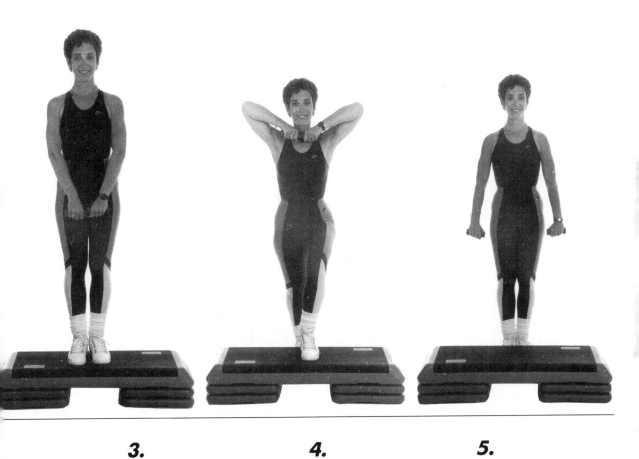

3.

Left foot steps up;
lower hands to the
original position.

4.

Right foot steps down;
raise the hands up to
the chin.

5.

Left foot steps down;
lower hands to the
original position.

18. Basic Step with Wide Rows

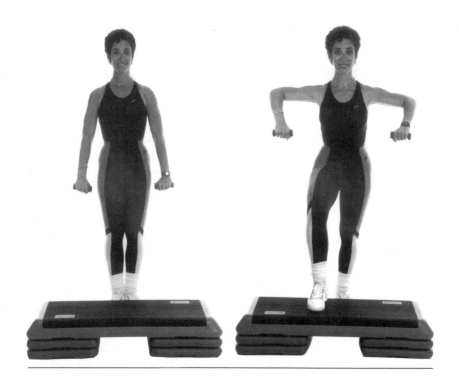

1.

Stand behind the step; arms are down by your sides.

2.

Right foot steps up; arms bend at ninety degrees at the elbows; lift arms up; squeeze back (shoulders are down).

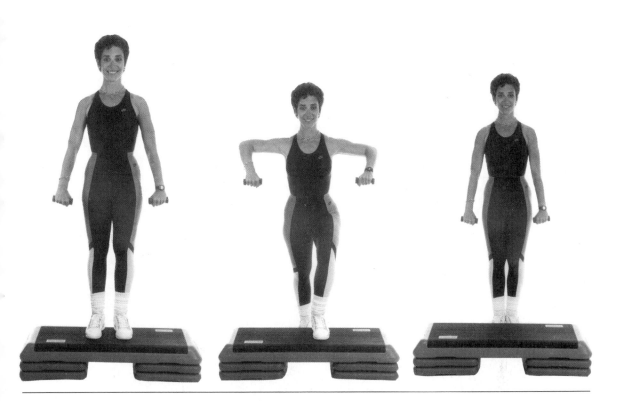

3.

Left foot steps up; press arms back down to the original position.

4.

Right foot steps down; arms bend at ninety degrees at the elbows; lift arms up; squeeze back (shoulders are down).

5.

Left foot steps down; lower arms down to the original position.

19. Mid-Range Latissimus Dorsi Pulls (Back Pulls)

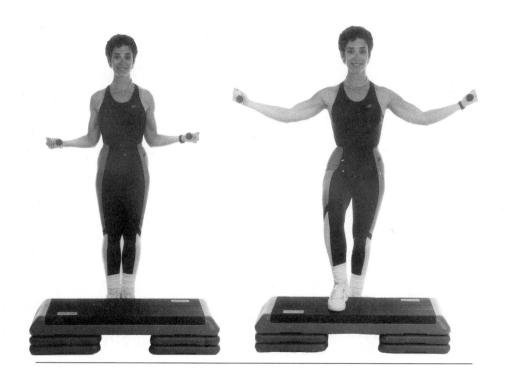

1.

Stand behind the step; arms are pinned in at the waist; elbows are at a ninety-degree angle.

2.

Right foot steps up; arms lift out at ninety degrees; elbows are bent.

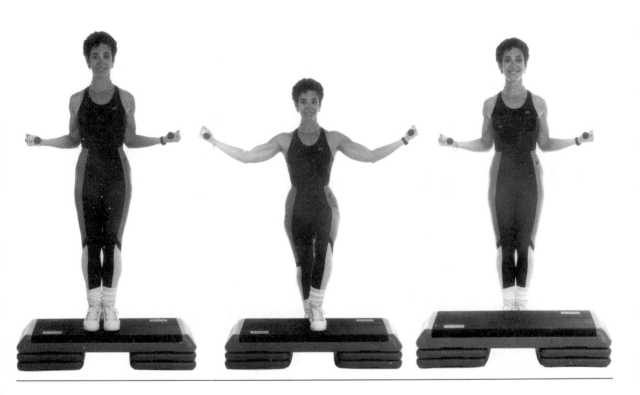

3.
Left foot steps up; arms are pinned in at the waist; elbows are at a ninety-degree angle; squeeze back.

4.
Right foot steps down; arms lift out again.

5.
Left foot steps down; arms return to the original position.

20. Upper Back Pulls

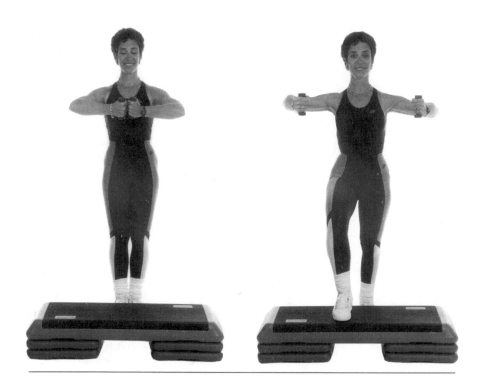

1.

Stand behind the step; elbows are out to the side; arms are in front of the chest with the hands pulled together.

2.

Right foot steps up; draw elbows back. You should feel your back squeezing; arms are chest height.

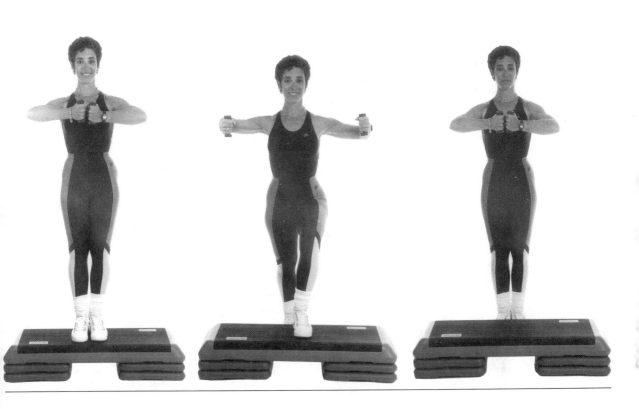

3.
Left foot steps up;
arms return to
beginning position.

4.
Right foot steps down;
draw elbows back,
chest height.

5.
Left foot steps down;
arms return to
beginning position.

21. Chest Flies

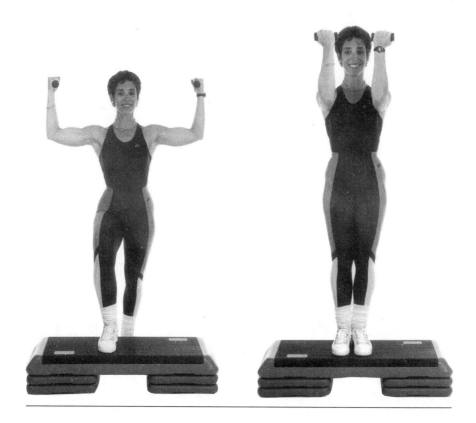

1.

Right foot steps up; arms are at ninety-degree angles; elbows are at shoulder height.

2.

Left foot steps up; arms pull in toward the chest, elbows lead; shoulders are down.

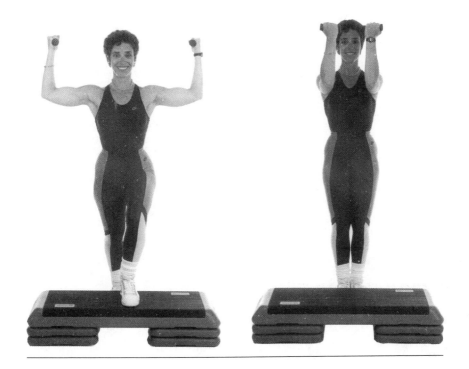

3.

Right foot steps down; arms go out again; elbows are at shoulder height.

4.

Left foot steps down; arms pull in toward the chest.

22. High-Range Shoulder Press

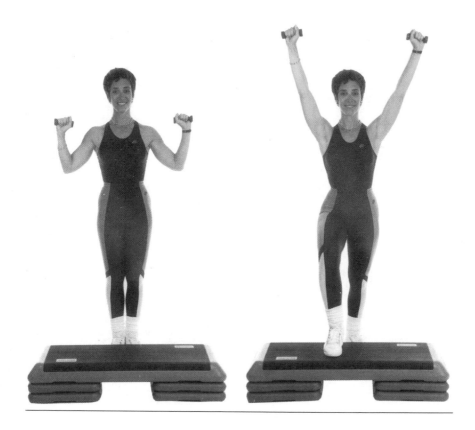

1.

Stand behind the step;
hands are at shoulder
height, elbows are bent,
palms face up.

2.

Right foot steps up;
arms push up overhead;
shoulders are down.

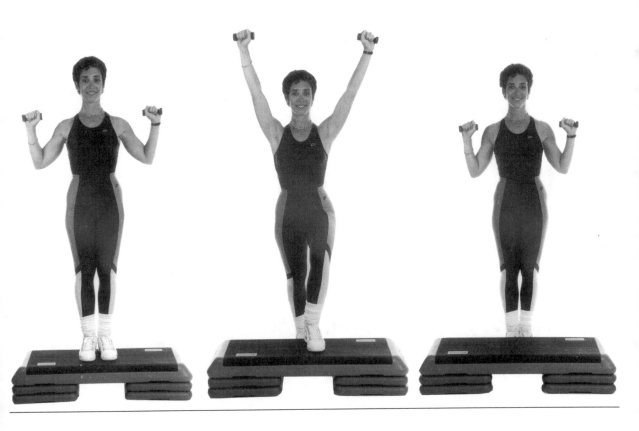

3.
Left foot steps up; hands return to shoulder height.

4.
Right foot steps down; arms push overhead.

5.
Left foot steps down; hands return to original position.

23. Wide Step

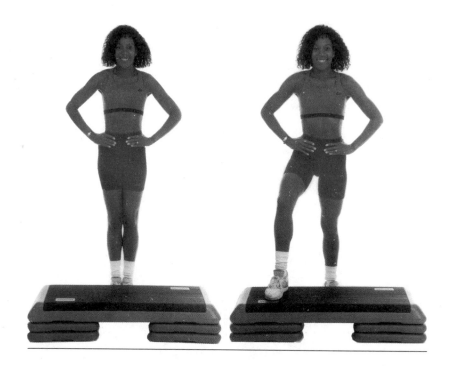

1.

Stand behind the step with your feet together; hands are on your hips.

2.

Right foot steps up as far to the right on the step as it can go without hanging off the edge (step wide).

Knees should only be slightly turned out.
Open your legs.

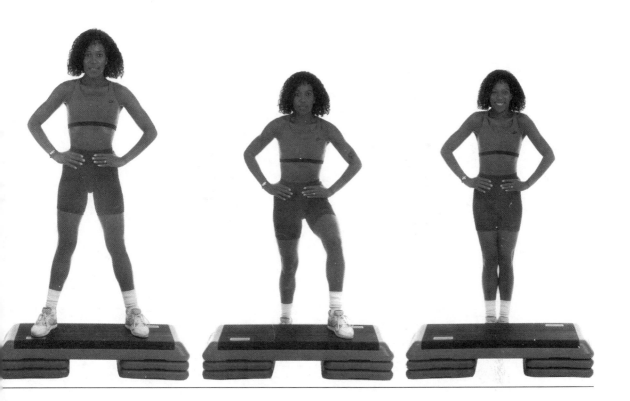

3.
Left foot steps up and wide.

4.
Right foot steps down behind the center of the step.

5.
Left foot steps down to meet the right foot.

24. **W**ide Step with Arm Extensions

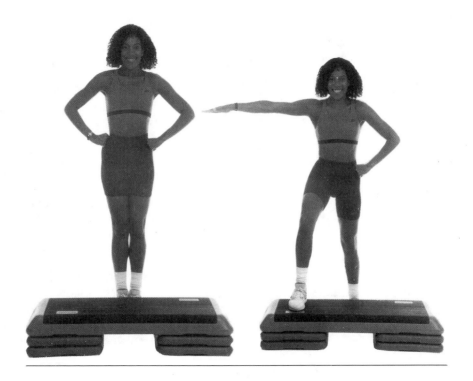

1.

Stand behind the step with your feet together; hands are on your hips.

2.

Right foot steps out and wide; right arm extends straight out to the side; left hand remains on hip.

Right arm follows right leg. Left arm follows left leg.

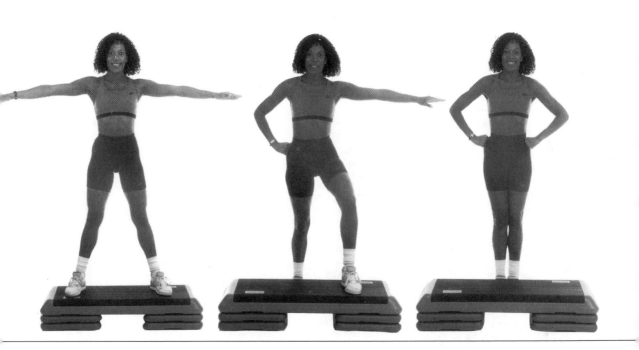

3.

Left foot steps out and wide; left arm extends straight out to the side.

4.

Right foot steps down; right hand returns to the hip.

5.

Left foot steps down; left hand returns to the hip.

25. Transition Step and Alternating Tap Step with Bicep Curls

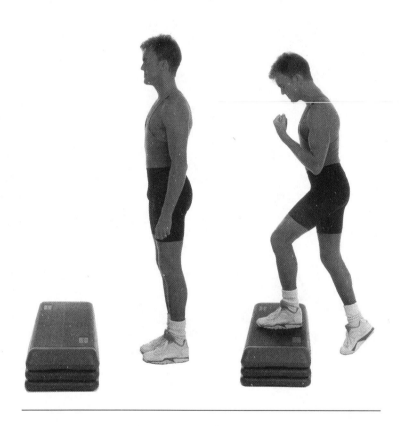

1.

Stand behind the step with feet together, arms down.

2.

Left foot steps up; arms curl up to chest level; squeeze the biceps.

3.

Right foot steps up; arms go down.

This exercise can be used to change leading foot after one minute or as an alternating step. All arm variations may be used.

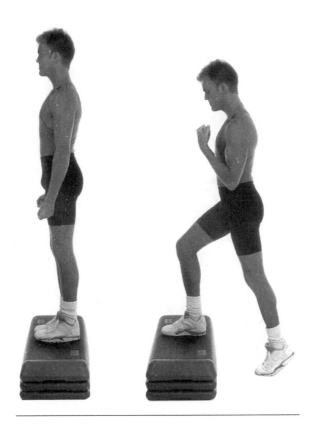

4.

Left foot steps down; arms curl up.

5.

Right foot taps down (tap is no weight on your foot); arms go down.

26. Turning Step

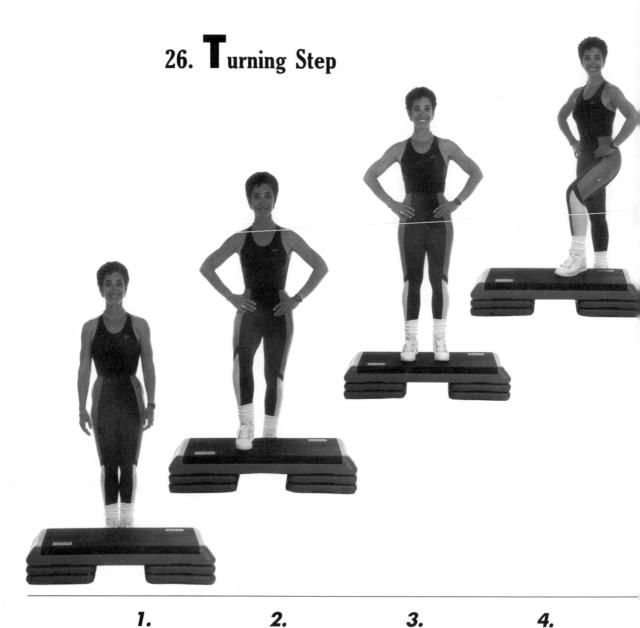

1.

Stand behind the step with arms down by your sides.

2.

Right foot steps up; put your hands on your hips.

3.

Left foot steps up; hands remain on your hips.

4.

Step down with right foot on a diagonal, hands on hips.

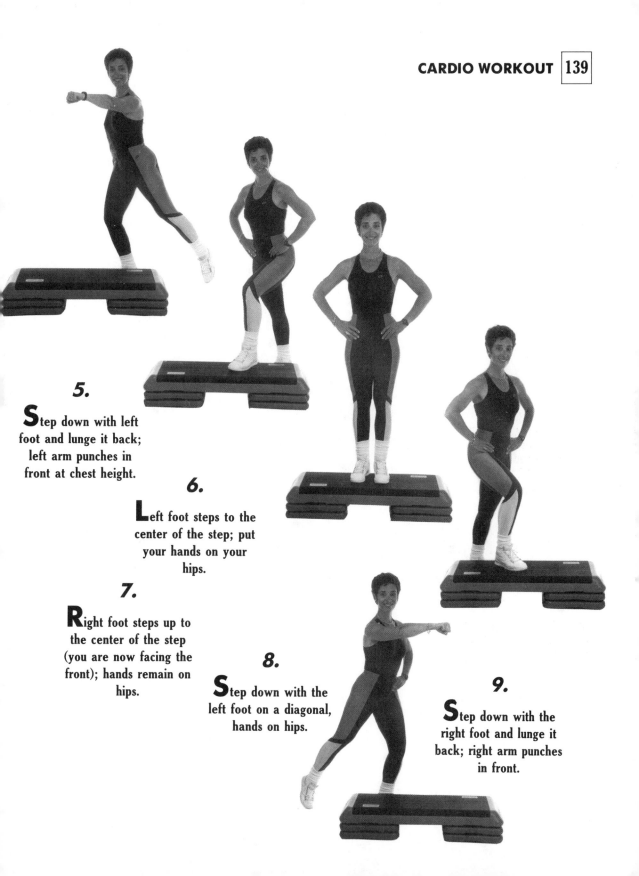

5.

Step down with left foot and lunge it back; left arm punches in front at chest height.

6.

Left foot steps to the center of the step; put your hands on your hips.

7.

Right foot steps up to the center of the step (you are now facing the front); hands remain on hips.

8.

Step down with the left foot on a diagonal, hands on hips.

9.

Step down with the right foot and lunge it back; right arm punches in front.

27. **K**nee Up/Tap Down

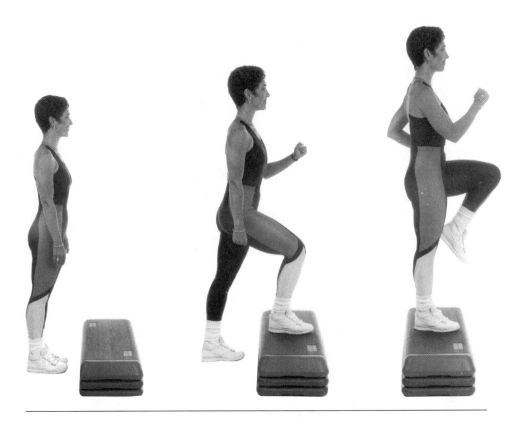

1.
Stand behind the step; arms are down.

2.
Right foot steps up; right arm is down; left arm lifts to hip level with a bent elbow.

3.
Left knee comes up; right leg is straight; right arm lifts to hip level with a bent elbow (as in a marching motion).

This step does not alternate. It uses the same leading leg.

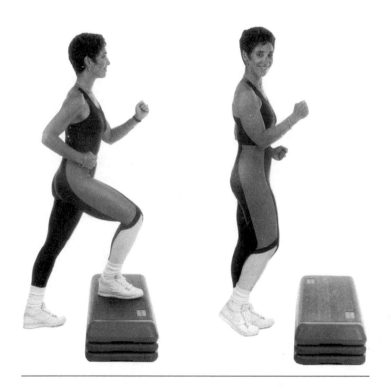

4.
Step down with the left leg; lift the left arm higher than the right arm.

5.
Tap down with the right foot.

28. **S**tep Knee Up
(alternating step)

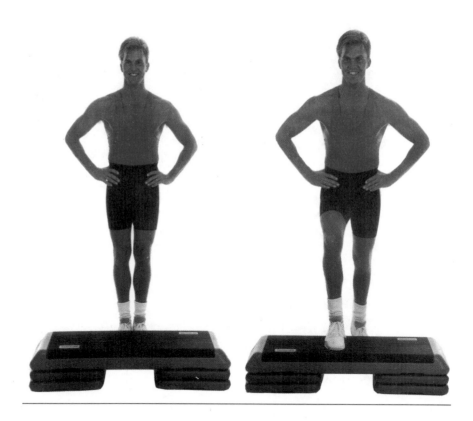

1.
Stand behind the step
with hands on hips.

2.
Right foot steps up;
hands remain on hips.

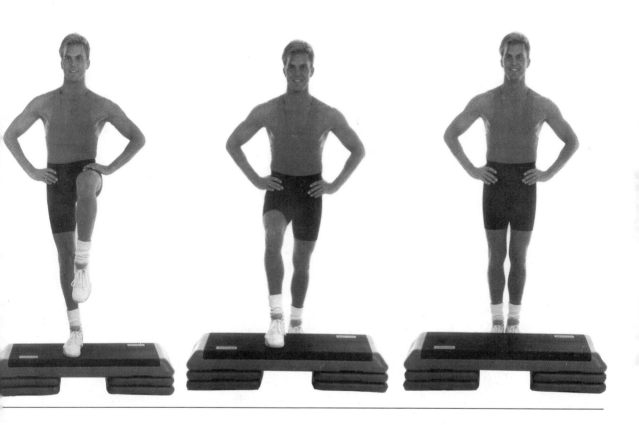

3.

Left knee comes up; right leg stays on the step.

4.

Left foot steps down.

5.

Right foot steps down.

29. Repeating Knee Lifts with Shoulder Press

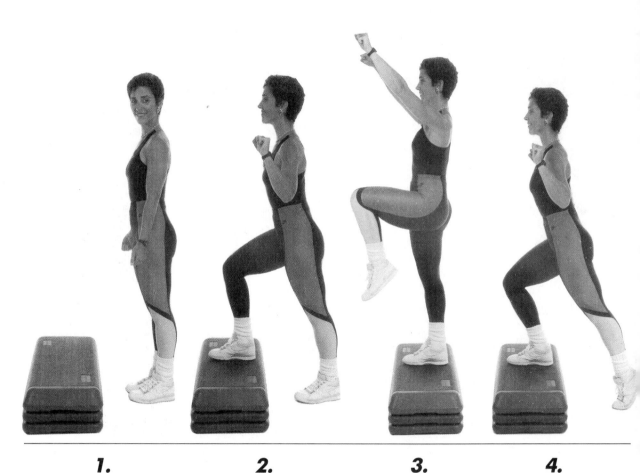

1.

Stand behind the step with your arms down by your sides.

2.

Right foot steps up; arms are at a ninety-degree angle near the shoulders.

3.

Left knee comes up; arms push overhead.

4.

Left foot taps down (only toe touches); arms go back to shoulder height.

Between knee lifts the foot goes back to the floor and touches. Keep all weight forward on the front foot and just touch the toe back. Eight counts.

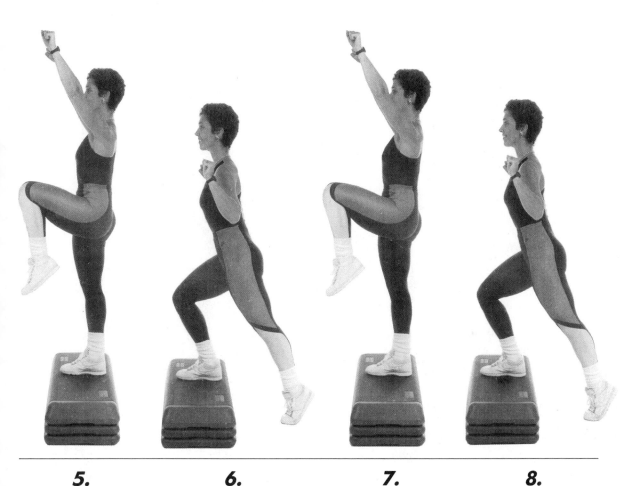

5.

Left knee comes back up; arms push overhead.

6.

Left foot taps down; arms go back to shoulder height.

7.

Left knee comes back up; arms push overhead.

8.

Left foot steps down; arms go back to shoulder height.

30. Turning Alternate Knee Lifts for Eight Counts

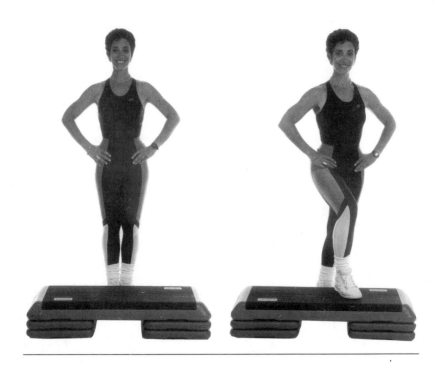

1.

Stand behind the step with your hands on your hips.

2.

Right foot steps up on a diagonal; hands remain on your hips.

3.

Left knee lifts up.

Inside foot, or foot closest to the step, steps first.

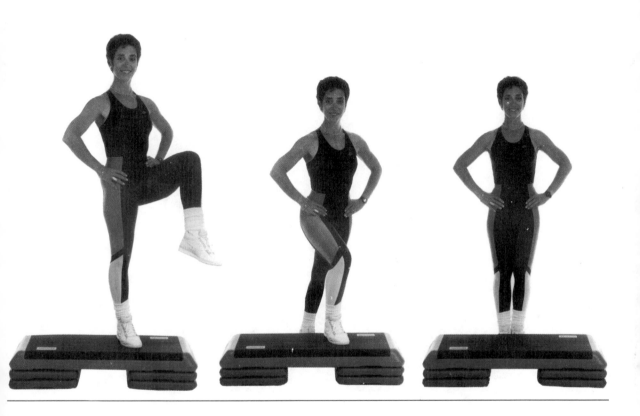

4.

Left foot steps down.

5.

Right foot steps down and faces center again.

6.

Repeat on the other side starting with the left foot.

31. Split Arm Variation for Turning with Alternating Knee Lifts

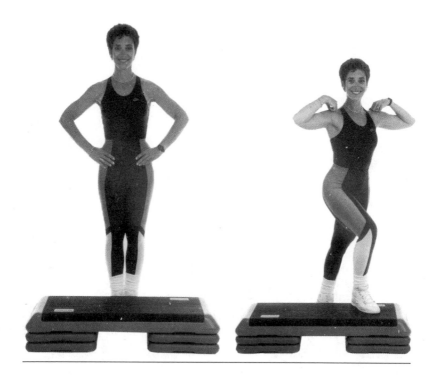

1.

Stand behind the step with your hands on your hips.

2.

Right foot steps up on a diagonal; put your hands on your shoulders.

3.

Left knee lifts up; right hand touches left calf.

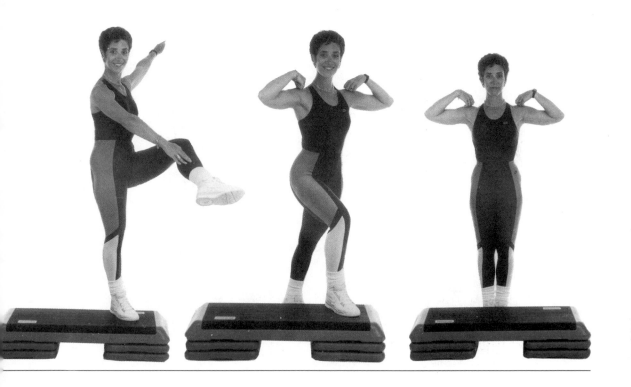

4.
Left foot steps down; hand returns to your shoulder.

5.
Right foot steps down on a diagonal; face the center of the step.

6.
Repeat starting with the left foot.

32. Heel Back with Split Arms

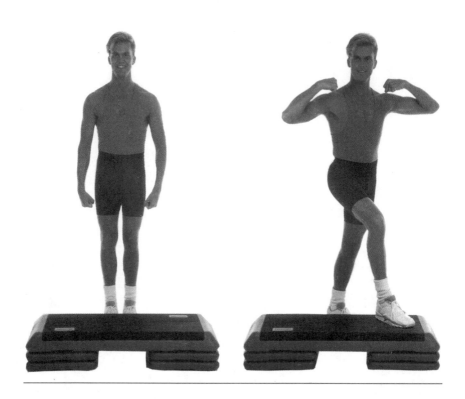

1.
Stand behind the step with your arms at your sides.

2.
Right foot steps up on a diagonal; put your hands on your shoulders.

3.
Left heel comes back; right arm touches the left heel; left arm shoots up and forward.

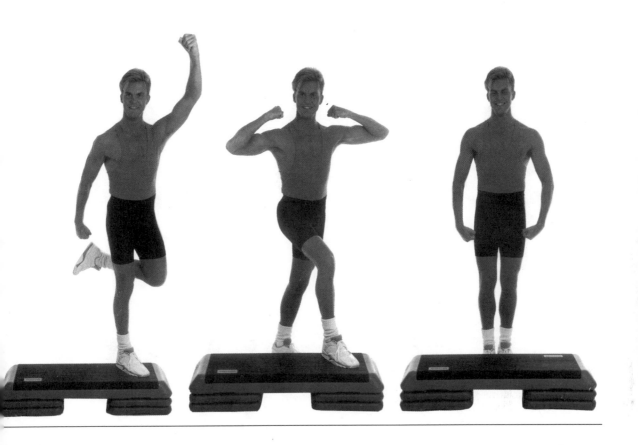

4.

Left leg returns to the floor; arms return to your shoulders.

5.

Right foot steps down on a diagonal; arms return to your sides.

6.

Repeat starting with the left foot.

33. Arabesque with Arms

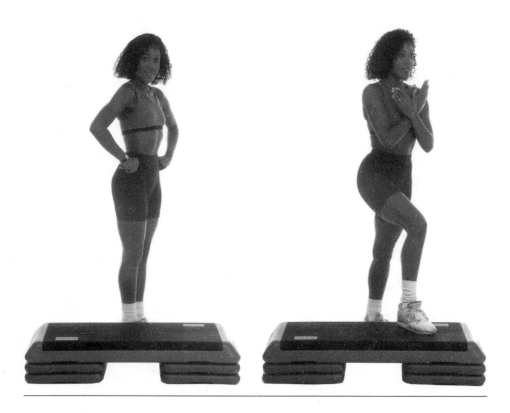

1.

Stand behind the step on a left diagonal; hands are on your hips.

2.

Right foot steps up on a right diagonal; arms cross at the chest; hands are up.

3.

Lean forward slightly and raise your left leg up and back (this is called an arabesque); right arm reaches straight out front; left arm extends down behind the buttock for balance).

When leg extends back, keep abdominals lifted. Draw leg back and squeeze the buttocks. Think of lifting up, not arching back.

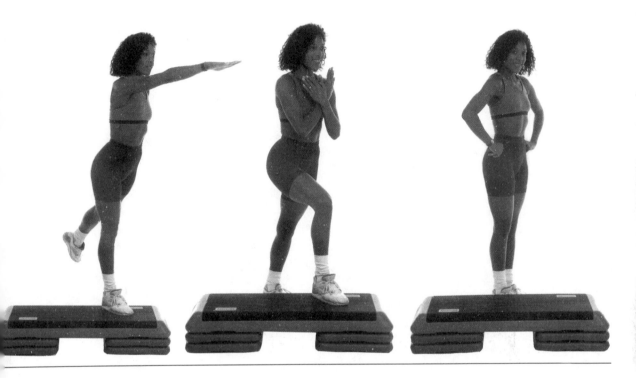

4.

Step down with the left foot; arms cross at the chest.

5.

Right foot steps down and faces center again; place hands on hips.

6.

Repeat starting with the left foot.

34. Basic Step from the End of the Step with Lateral Press

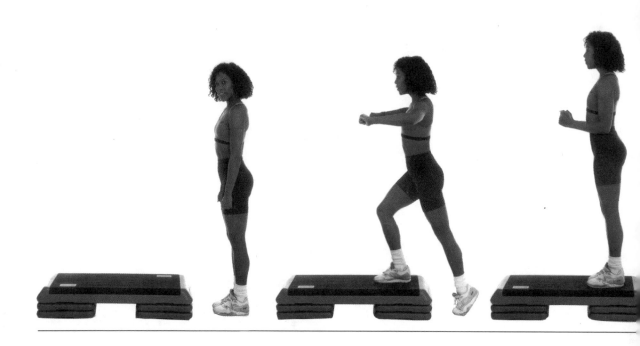

1.

Stand at one end of the step with legs together; arms are down.

2.

Right foot steps up onto the end of the step; arms come out to the side at shoulder height; elbows are bent.

3.

Left foot steps up; arms come in to the waist; thumbs face up.

You may do any type of arm variation with this exercise.

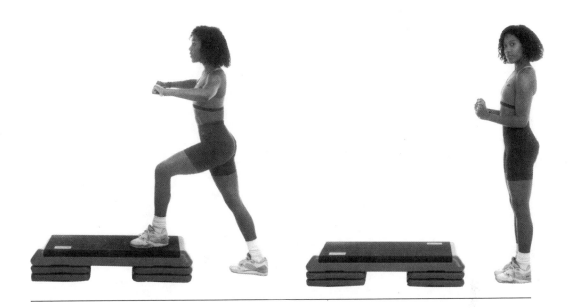

4.

Right foot steps down; arms come up again.

5.

Left foot steps down; arms come in to the waist.

35. **A**lternate Knee Lift from the End of the Step with Chest Push

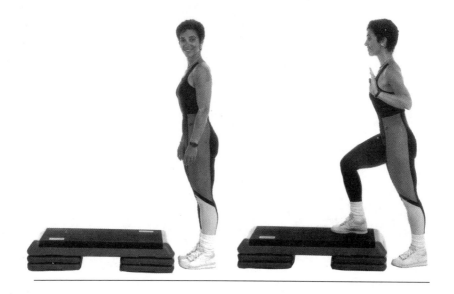

1.

Stand at the left end of the step, feet together; arms are down at your sides.

2.

Right foot steps up; arms come up by the chest; hands face out.

Any arm variations are possible in this exercise.

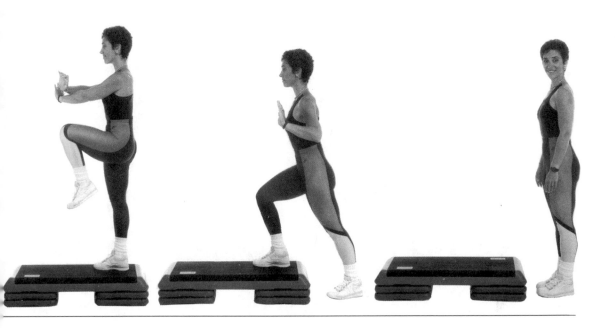

3.
Left knee lifts up; arms push out in front of the chest.

4.
Left foot steps down; arms return to the chest position.

5.
Right foot steps down; hands return to your sides.

36. Squats Off the End of the Step (may also be performed facing front)

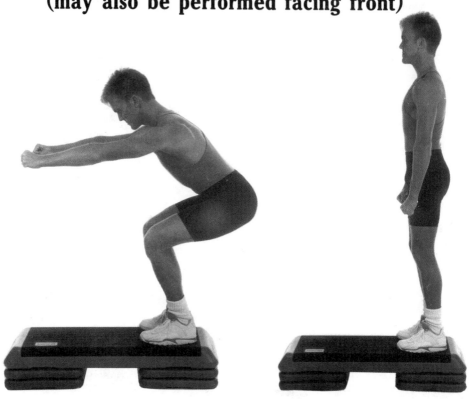

1.

Stand on the end of the step. Sit back with your chest up; knees are over the center of the foot, the body weight is over the top half of the thighs; reach forward for two counts.

2.

Push up, using the legs and buttocks, to standing position for two counts.

3.

Repeat sequence eight times.

37. Lunges Off the End of the Step
(may also be performed facing front)

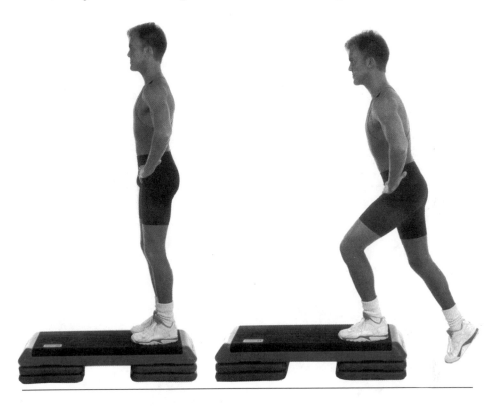

1.

Stand on the end of the step with your feet together; hands are on your hips.

2.

Right leg taps down; hands remain on your hips.

3.

Right foot steps up; hands are still on your hips.

4.

Repeat starting with the left leg.

> **Keep your knee over the center of your foot. Your body should be lifted and the weight should be on the forward foot.**

38. Over the Top
(alternating eight counts)

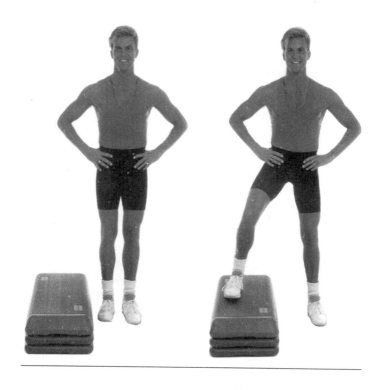

1.
Begin on the left side of the step; hands are on your hips where they will remain.

2.
Right foot steps up.

You travel from one side of the step to the other. All arm variations are possible in this exercise.

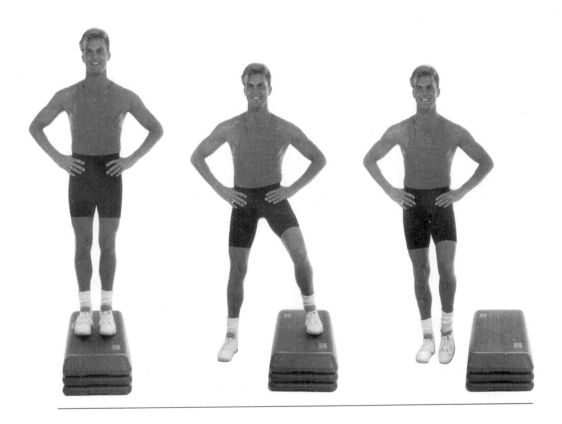

3.
Left foot steps up.

4.
Right foot steps forward and down (you are now on the other side of the step).

5.
Left foot taps down.

6.
Repeat leading with the left foot.

39. Over the Top with Lateral Shoulder Raises

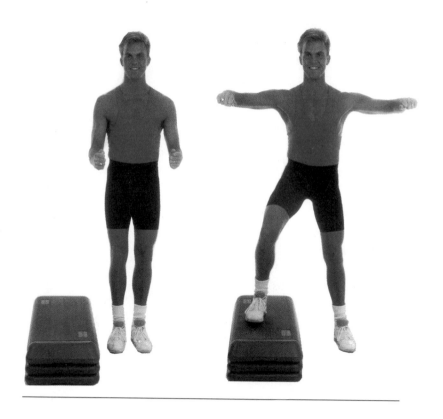

1.

Stand on the left side of the step; arms are lifted up by your waist; elbows are bent.

2.

Right foot steps up; arms lift out at shoulder height to the side.

3.

Left foot steps up; arms return to your waist.

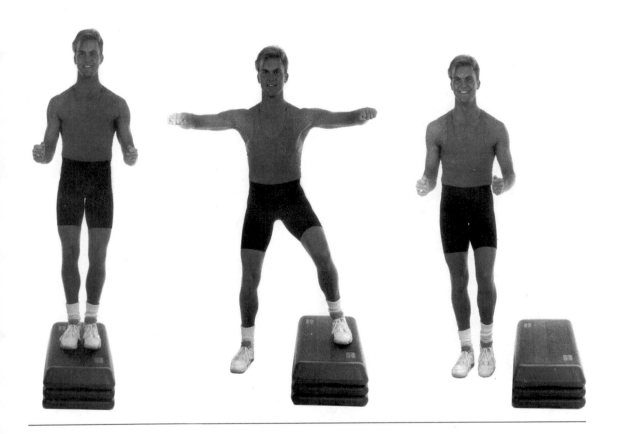

4.

Right foot steps down; arms lift out at shoulder height to the side.

5.

Left foot taps down; arms return to your waist.

6.

Repeat.

40. Tap Up/Tap Down

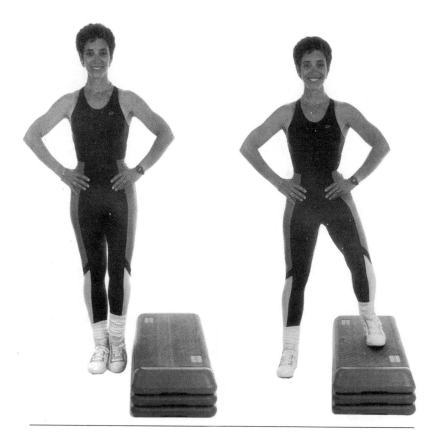

1.
Stand on the right side of the step; hands are on your hips where they will remain.

2.
Left foot steps up.

All arm variations are possible in this exercise. You may also raise your knee up with the second leg for another variation (i.e., right foot up, left knee up, left foot down, right foot taps down).

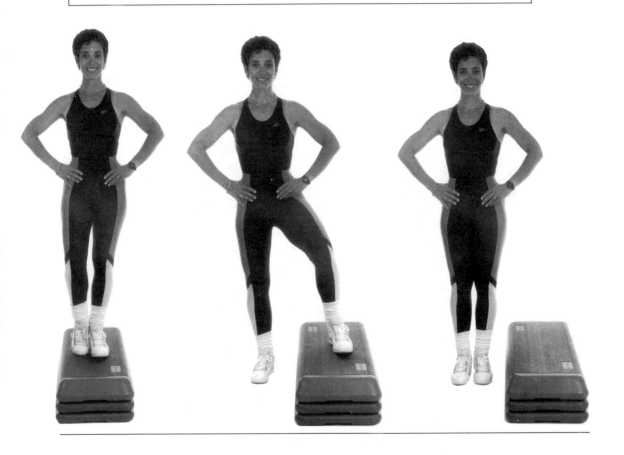

3.
Right foot taps up.

4.
Right foot steps down.

5.
Left foot taps down.

41. Straddle Up

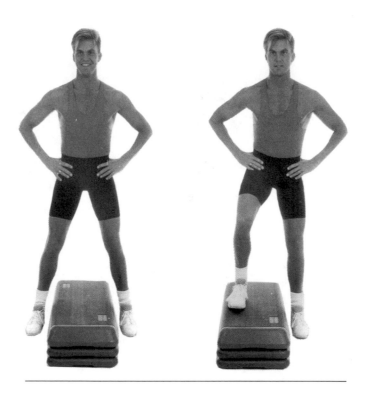

1.

Begin by straddling the step—feet are on either side of the step; hands are on hips throughout this exercise.

2.

Right foot steps up.

You may alternate by tapping down on the last step.
All arm variations are possible.

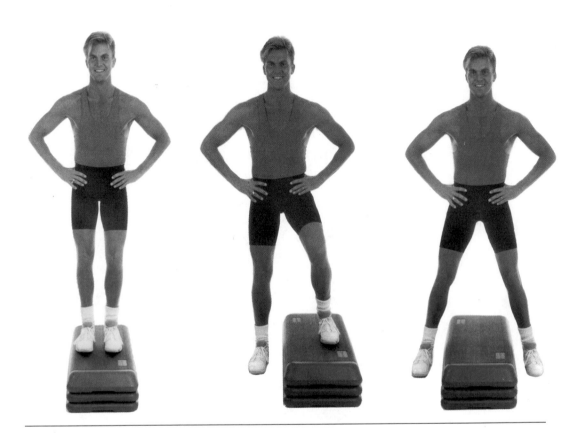

3.
Left foot steps up.

4.
Right foot steps down.

5.
Left foot steps down.

42. **S**traddle Up with Low Back Pull

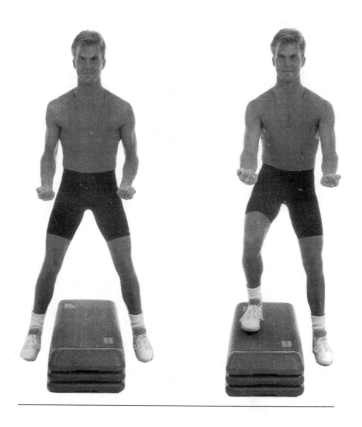

1.

Straddle the step with your arms at waist height; elbows are pulled in.

2.

Right foot steps up; reach your arms forward, palms up.

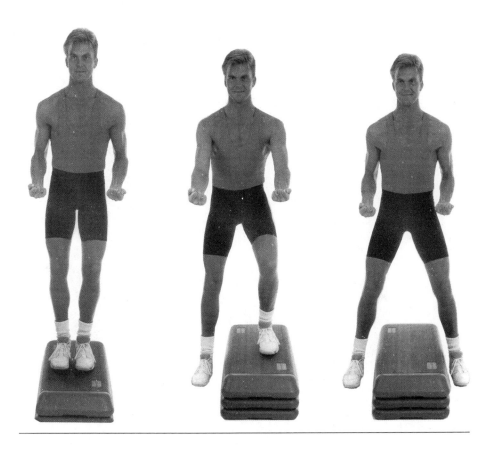

3.

Left foot steps up; pull elbows back again.

4.

Right foot steps down (over the top); reach arms forward.

5.

Left foot steps down; elbows are pinned back.

43. Straddle Knee Up, Alternating with Double Low Jabs for Eight Counts

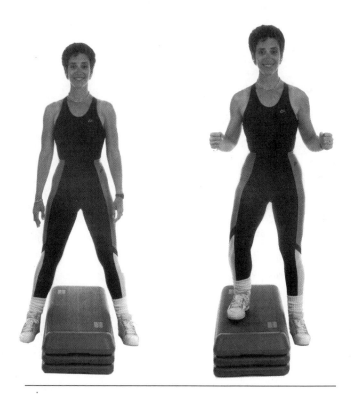

1.
Straddle the step; arms are down by your sides.

2.
Right foot steps up; elbows are pulled in by the waist at ninety degrees, palms facing each other.

3.
Pull the left knee up; cross forearms in front.

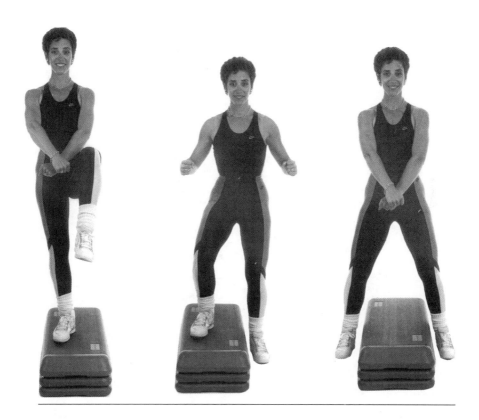

4.

Left foot steps down; arms are back to position 2.

5.

Right foot steps down (back to straddle position); arms cross in front.

6.

Repeat starting with the left leg.

44. **S**traddle Down

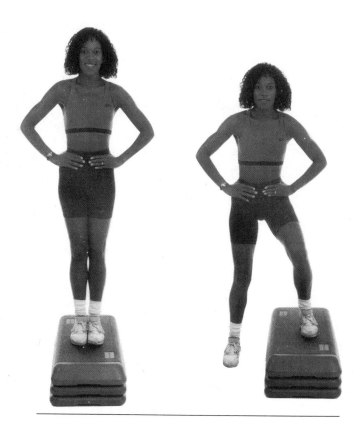

1.

Begin on top of the step; hands are on the waist where they will remain.

2.

Right foot steps down; left foot remains on the top of the step.

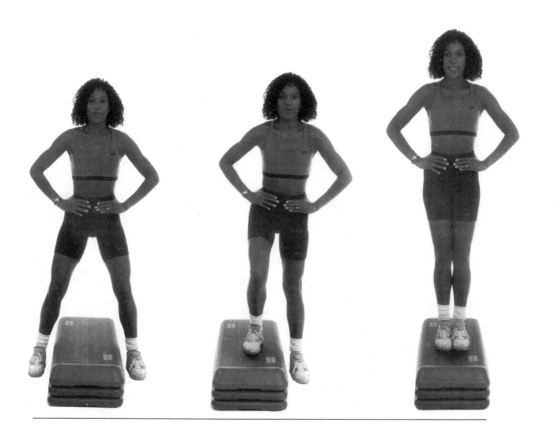

3.

Left foot steps down
(you are now straddling
the step).

4.

Right foot steps up.

5.

Left foot steps up.

45. Straddle Down with Knee Up and Chest Flies

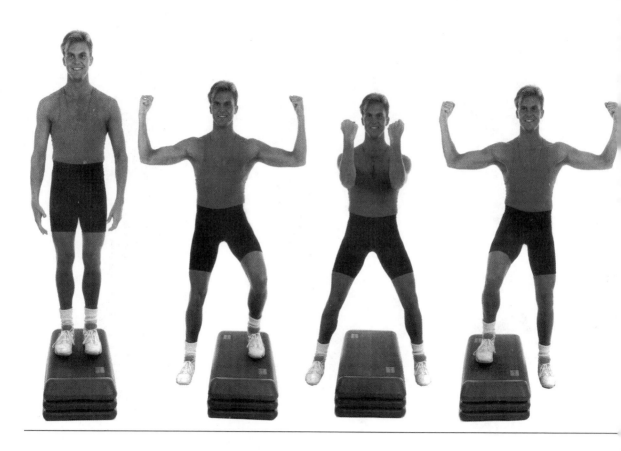

1.

Stand on top of the step with your arms by your sides.

2.

Right foot steps down; arms open at ninety degrees with elbows bent.

3.

Left foot steps down (straddle position); arms pull in front of your face.

4.

Right foot steps up; arms bend open again.

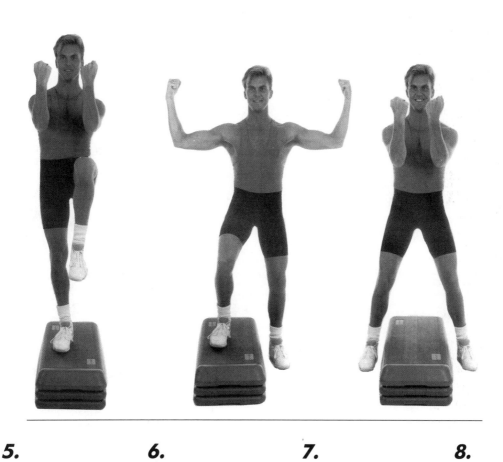

5.

Left knee lifts up; arms pull in front of your face.

6.

Left foot steps down; arms open.

7.

Right foot steps down (straddle position); arms pull in.

8.

Repeat with the left foot stepping down first, right knee lifting up.

46. Lunges

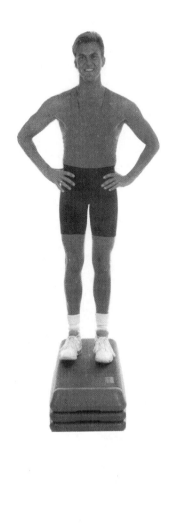
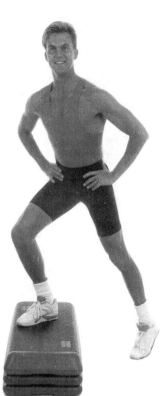

1.

Stand on the top of the step; hands are on your hips where they will remain.

2.

Lunge back with your left foot (diagonally off the step), only the toe touches the floor (no weight on toe).

3.

Left foot returns to the top of the step.

4.

Repeat lunging with the right foot.

Keep your knee over the center of your foot. Weight should be on the forward foot.

47. Lunges with Different Arm Variations

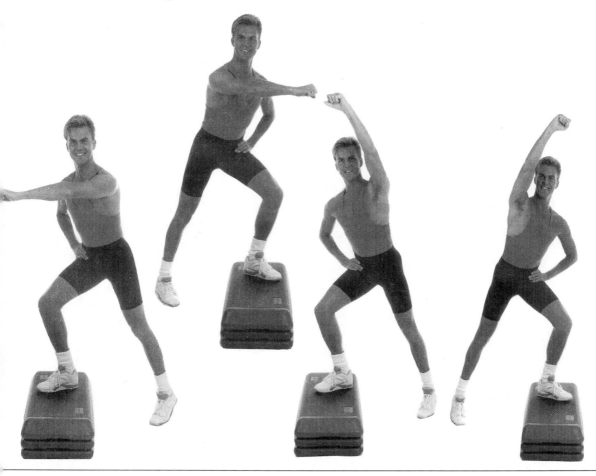

1.

Lunge back with your left foot; left arm reaches across your chest; hand is in a fist.

2.

Lunge back with your right foot; right arm punches across your chest.

3.

Left foot lunges back; left arm reaches up; hand is in a fist.

4.

Right foot lunges back; right arm reaches up; hand is in a fist.

Proceed to cool-down stretches.

SAMPLE WORKOUTS

Here are several customized Step On It workouts, using the exercises from the book. Feel free to put together your own workout combinations as well. Don't forget to do a warm-up before you start and a cool down when you are finished.

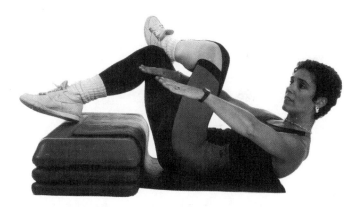

Sample Aerobic Step On It Workouts

1. (Ten minutes, one minute equals thirty, four-count cycles)

1 minute   Basic Step, right foot leads with Bicep Curls

1 minute   Basic Step, left foot leads with Tricep Extensions

1 minute   Basic Step, right foot leads with Alternate Bicep Curls

1 minute   Basic Step, left foot leads with Alternate Hammer Curls

1 minute   Alternating Tap Step with Shoulder Raises

1 minute   Wide Step, right foot leads with Arm Extensions

1 minute   Wide Step, left foot leads with Arm Extensions

1 minute   Alternating Wide Tap Step with Alternating Arm Extensions

1 minute   Alternating Step Knee Up, *no arms*

1 minute   Alternating Step Knee Up with Shoulder Press

2. (Ten minutes; you may combine with above for a twenty-minute workout)

1 minute   Basic Step, right foot leads with Chest Flies

1 minute   Basic Step, left foot leads with Back Pulls

1 minute   Alternating Tap Step with Alternating Bicep Curls

1 minute   Alternating Turning Step with Alternating Bicep Curls

1 minute   Alternating Over the Top Step with Alternating Bicep Curls
End one-minute segment on the same side of step you started
on.

1 minute   Knee Up/Tap Down, right leg leads with Natural Arms

1 minute   Basic Step, right foot leads with Rear Shoulder Lifts

1 minute   Basic Step, left foot leads with Crisscross Arms

3. (Ten minutes; you may combine with all of the above for a thirty-
minute workout)

Begin by standing on the top of the step facing one end.
1 minute   Straddle off the step, right foot leads with Alternating Bicep
            Curls. After 1 minute use a tap transition.

1 minute   Straddle off the step, left foot leads with Alternating Bicep
            Curls

1 minute   Straddle off the step, Knee Lifts with Alternating Bicep Curls
            (down, down, up, knee)

1 minute   Squats, off the back end, two times for eight counts, followed
            by four lunges for eight counts

1 minute   Basic Step off the back end, right foot leads with Front
            Shoulder Raises

1 minute   Basic Step off the back end, left foot leads with Shoulder Rotations

Begin the next sequence by straddling the step.

1 minute   Straddle on, right foot leads with Shoulder Raises

1 minute   Straddle off, left foot leads with Shoulder Presses

1 minute   Lunges, off the side of the step, alternate right foot and left foot; extend right arm in front when right foot lunges and left arm in front when left foot lunges

1 minute   Alternating Tap Step, off the back end with Reverse Bicep Curls

---

For information on purchasing step training equipment, please call 1-800-STAY-STEP or 1-800-25-BENCH.